Communications in Computer and Information Science   975

Commenced Publication in 2007
Founding and Former Series Editors:
Phoebe Chen, Alfredo Cuzzocrea, Xiaoyong Du, Orhun Kara, Ting Liu,
Krishna M. Sivalingam, Dominik Ślęzak, and Xiaokang Yang

More information about this series at http://www.springer.com/series/7899

Jan Cabri · Pedro Pezarat-Correia ·
João Vilas-Boas (Eds.)

Sport Science Research and Technology Support

4th and 5th International Congress, icSPORTS 2016
Porto, Portugal, November 7–9, 2016, and icSPORTS 2017
Funchal, Madeira, Portugal, October 30–31, 2017
Revised Selected Papers

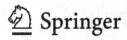 Springer

Editors
Jan Cabri
Norwegian School of Sport Sciences
Oslo, Norway

Pedro Pezarat-Correia
Universidade de Lisboa
Cruz Quebrada, Portugal

João Vilas-Boas
Faculty of Sport, and Porto Biomechanics
University of Porto
Porto, Portugal

ISSN 1865-0929   ISSN 1865-0937   (electronic)
Communications in Computer and Information Science
ISBN 978-3-030-14525-5   ISBN 978-3-030-14526-2   (eBook)
https://doi.org/10.1007/978-3-030-14526-2

Library of Congress Control Number: 2019932789

This Springer imprint is published by the registered company Springer Nature Switzerland AG
The registered company address is: Gewerbestrasse 11, 6330 Cham, Switzerland

Preface

In the twenty-first century most human activities, including sports, are becoming more and more technological. Engineering in general and information technology in particular are becoming an important support for many activities directly or indirectly related to sport sciences, including improvement of physical activities, sports medicine, biotechnology and nutrition, sports management, and all imaginable application areas in sports.

The present book includes extended and revised versions of a set of selected papers from the International Congress on Sport Sciences Research and Technology Support, icSPORTS 2016 and 2017 editions. These congresses were intended to be a meeting point for both academics and practitioners from different technological areas to exchange ideas and develop synergies.

icSPORTS 2016 received 53 paper submissions from 25 countries, of which 11% are included in this book.

icSPORTS 2017 received 40 paper submissions from 19 countries, of which 15% are included in this book.

The papers were selected by the event chairs and their selection is based on several criteria including the classifications and comments provided by the Program Committee members, the session chairs' assessment, and the program chairs' global view of all papers included in the technical program. The authors of selected papers were then invited to submit a revised and extended version of their papers having at least 30% innovative material.

The papers selected in this book contribute to the understanding of relevant trends of current research in technology support applied to sport sciences in areas such as training and testing, health and fitness, or sport biomechanics. New ideas and technical developments are presented in simulation and mathematical modeling, in computer-supported training and decision support systems, or in multimedia and information technology.

We would like to thank all the authors for their contributions and also the reviewers who helped ensure the quality of this publication.

November 2017

Jan Cabri
Pedro Pezarat-Correia
João Vilas-Boas

Organization

Conference Chair

Jan Cabri   Norwegian School of Sport Sciences, Norway

Co-chairs

Pedro Pezarat-Correia   Universidade de Lisboa, Portugal
João Vilas-Boas   University of Porto, Portugal

Program Committee

Served in 2016

Abdülkerim Baltaci	Selçuk University, Medical Faculty, Turkey
Benedicte Vanwanseele	KU Leuven, Belgium
Carl Payton	Manchester Metropolitan University, UK
Christos Spitas	Delft University of Technology, The Netherlands
Conor Gissane	Saint Mary's University College Twickenham, UK
Dafna Merom	University of Western Sydney, Australia
Daniel Boullosa	Universidade Católica de Brasília, Brazil
Daniel James	Griffith University, Australia
David Rowlands	Griffith University, Australia
David Thiel	Griffith University, Australia
David Whiteside	USA
Doug King	Hutt Valley District Health Board, New Zealand
Federico Schena	University of Verona, Italy
François Hug	The University of Queensland, Australia
Gary Brickley	University of Brighton, UK
Glyn Howatson	University of Northumbria, UK
Hayri Ertan	Anadolu University, Turkey
Helena Santa-Clara	Universidade de Lisboa, Portugal
Hermann Schwameder	Salzburg University, Austria
John Challis	The Pennsylvania State University, USA
Kane Middleton	La Trobe University, Australia
Karl-Peter Benedetto	Landeskrankenhause Feldkirch, Austria
Keith Lyons	University of Canberra, Australia
Kerstin Witte	Otto von Guericke University Magdeburg, Germany
Marco Cardinale	Aspire Academy, Qatar
Matthew Pain	Loughborough University, UK
Michael Grey	University of Birmingham, UK
Nelson Cortes	George Mason University, USA

Nicola Lai   Old Dominion University, USA
Oliver Faude   University of Basel, Switzerland
Orlando Fernandes   Universidade de Évora, Portugal
Patria Hume   Auckland University of Technology, New Zealand
Rita Cordovil   Universidade Técnica de Lisboa, Portugal
Terry Haggerty   University of New Brunswick, Canada
Walery Zukow   Kazimierz Wielki University, Poland

Served in 2017

Ali Shaifnezhad   Sports Sciences Research Institute of Iran,
                              Iran, Islamic Republic of
Andrew Kilding   Auckland University of Technology, New Zealand
Anthony Leicht   James Cook University, Australia
Antoine Nordez   University of Nantes, France
Aurélien Pichon   Université de Poitiers, France
David Cabello   Manrique Universidad de Granada, Spain
Giuseppe D'Antona   University of Pavia, Italy
Hannah Wyatt   Cardiff Metropolitan University, UK
Kirsti Uusi-Rasi   UKK Institute for Health Promotion Research, Finland
Luís Silva   Universidade Lusiada, Portugal
Maria Castro   Health School of Coimbra - IPC, Portugal
Sebahattin Devecioglu   Firat University, Turkey

Served in 2016 and 2017

Alessandro Pezzoli   Politecnico di Torino and Università di Torino, Italy
Andreia Sousa   Instituto Politécnico do Porto, Portugal
Andrey Koptyug   Mid Sweden University, Sweden
Arnold Baca   University of Vienna, Austria
Cathy Craig   Queen's University Belfast, UK
Chris Mills   University of Portsmouth, UK
Fernando Diefenthaeler   Universidade Federal de Santa Catarina, Brazil
Fernando Ribeiro   Universidade de Aveiro, Portugal
Floren Colloud   Université de Poitiers, France
Franco Impellizzeri   University of Technology of Sydney, Australia
Gregoire Millet   Institute of Sports Sciences, University of Lausanne,
                              Switzerland
Hans Weghorn   BW Cooperative State University Stuttgart, Germany
Henrique Jones   Clínica Ortopédica do Montijo, Portugal
Herbert Ugrinowitsch   Universidade Federal de Minas Gerais, Brazil
Jan Cabri   Norwegian School of Sport Sciences, Norway
José Barela   Universidade Cruzeiro do Sul, Brazil
José Faria   Universidade da Beira Interior, Portugal
José Pereira   Escola Superior de Tecnologia de Setúbal, Portugal
Kazumoto Tanaka   Kindai University, Japan
Laura Capranica   Università degli Studi di Roma Foro Italico, Italy

Luis Espejo Antúnez	Extremadura University, Spain
Marianne Gittoes	Cardiff Metropolitan University, UK
Mark Willems	University of Chichester, UK
Nuno Cordeiro	Escola Superior de Saúde Dr. Lopes Dias do Instituto Politécnico de Castelo Branco, Portugal
Pedro Pezarat-Correia	Universidade de Lisboa, Portugal
Peter Federolf	University of Innsbruck, Institute of Sport Science, Austria
Raul Oliveira	Universidade de Lisboa, Portugal
Rodrigo Bini	Universidade Federal do Rio Grande do Sul, Brazil
Ronaldo Gabriel	University of Trás-os-Montes and Alto Douro, Portugal
Rui Torres	North Polytechnic Institute of Health, Paredes, Portugal
Silvio Lorenzetti	Swiss Federal Institute of Sport Magglingen SFISM, Switzerland
Timothy Exell	University of Portsmouth, UK
Vasileios Exadaktylos	BioRICS, Belgium

Invited Speakers

2016

Jim Richards	Allied Health Research Unit, University of Central Lancashire, UK
Carlo Capelli	Norwegian School of Sport Sciences, Norway
Andy Harland	Loughborough University, UK

2017

Andrey Koptyug	Mid Sweden University, Sweden
Andreas Mierau	International University of Health, Exercise and Sports (LU:NEX), Luxembourg
Gert-Peter Brüggemann	Institute of Biomechanics and Orthopaedics, German Sport University Cologne, Germany

Contents

The Determinants of a Good Lunge Performance in Fencing - In Two Approaches

Carla P. Guimarães[1]([✉]), Vitor Balbio[1], Gloria L. Cid[1],
Maria Isabel V. Orselli[3], Ana Paula Xavier[1], Augusto Siqueira Neto[2],
and Sônia C. Corrêa[2]

[1] National Institute of Technology, Rio de Janeiro, Rio de Janeiro, Brazil
carla.guimaraes@int.gov.br
[2] LACEM, Presbyteriam University Mackenzie, Barueri, São Paulo, Brazil
[3] Franciscan University, Santa Maria, Rio Grande do Sul, Brazil

Abstract. A Lunge is the basis of most attacking motions in fencing. Several studies have tried to determine biomechanical parameters that are determinants for a good lunge performance by comparing the kinematics of lunge gesture in novice versus experienced fencers. The purpose of this study was to 1 - understand if there are biomechanical parameters common to a group of experienced athletes that are determinant for a good lunge performance and 2 - build a 3D platform to facilitate the visualization and interaction between biomechanical information and coaches. Five skilled épée fencing athletes had their marker trajectories captured with an OptiTrack digital motion system (Prime 13) using eighteen cameras. The subjects executed the lunge 5–6 times while the coach qualitatively evaluated their performance. The two best (BR) and the two worst (WR) rated trials of each athlete, according to coach criteria, were used in our analysis. Wilcoxon test showed no significant differences in any of the selected variables when comparing the BR and WR trials. Our results also indicated that the body position at front-foot heel contact can possibly be a particularly important determinant to lunge performance and that the 3D platform can help the coach visualize and understand this phase.

Keywords: Fencing · 3D digital platform · Kinematics

1 Introduction

Fencing is a result of speed and accuracy derived from a good skill, and this can be well evaluated with Biomechanics. A well defined movement pattern can be responsible for the athlete to reach the target faster and with less need of power. Lunge is the basis of most attacking motions in fencing and thus a well-executed gesture can be determinant to attack success. Several studies have tried to determine biomechanical parameters that are determinants for a good lunge performance by comparing the kinematics of lunge gesture in novice versus experienced fencers.

Using this approach [1] analyzed several factors that can influence lunge performance and observed that one of them was the center of mass (CM) potential energy, which decreases monotonically in the more skilled athletes, suggesting a link between

© Springer Nature Switzerland AG 2019
J. Cabri et al. (Eds.): icSPORTS 2016/2017, CCIS 975, pp. 1–17, 2019.
https://doi.org/10.1007/978-3-030-14526-2_1

coordination and skill. In a lunge, good coordination between the velocity changes that happen in the lower limbs motion, specially in the front leg, is essential to ensure an efficient conversion of potential into kinetic energy. Not surprisingly, it has been shown to affect the lunge and the weapon velocity and discriminate between novice and experienced fencers [2], to be an important element for the lunge performance.

There is a common belief described by [3] that during a lunge performance the weapon arm should move ahead of the body center of mass, nevertheless [2, 4] described that both movements can happen simultaneously.

In relation to predictors of the lunge motion [5] identified that knee range of motion, and peak hip flexion of the trailing leg and peak hip flexion of the leading leg were significant predictors of sword velocity and [6] found a significant correlation between lunge velocity and time to peak angular velocity of the trailing knee and leading elbow.

The authors in general are worried about the generation of the velocity and a few numbers of papers are found related to the kinematics chain, studying how the velocity is transferred. [7] described, using electromyography and kinematics data, that the trailing leg extensor muscles activate following a temporal pattern with the plantar flexors in the ankle firing subsequently. [8] found that expert fencing athletes demonstrated a sequential pattern from proximal to distal sequence in the trailing leg which was not as evident in the novices. Our group [9] showed the importance of the unarmed arm, as an auxiliary to the sword velocity and for the body stability.

In the present study, we ought to explore further the biomechanical factors that can affect the proper achievement of this sportive gesture in order to understand if there are biomechanical parameters common to a group of experienced athletes that are determinant for a good lunge performance.

Differently from previous studies, our approach took, primarily, into account the judgment of the individual performance established by an experienced coach. It is interesting to appoint that there is a big gap between scientific knowledge and coaches. Which take place all over the world. There is much knowledge being developed in labs however it never reaches the coaches. The languages are very different. The coach usually does not understand the graphics and data that the biomechanic researchers generate and the coaches need something that they can really use in their daily practice.

We intend to work in this gap, trying to fill the coaches' needs but bringing the precision and reliable data that we can provide. The use of an interactive system is interesting and can fill this gap communication between coaches' and researchers. The Ergonomic Laboratory researchers of the National Institute of Technology [10] have been working on this approach in other projects that involve combat sports such as Jiu-jitu and also in ergonomic study applied to the education and training of caregivers.

The purpose of this research is to understand if there are biomechanical parameters common to a group of experienced athletes that are determinant for a good lunge performance in accordance to a coach criteria and build a 3D digital platform to facilitate the visualization and interaction between biomechanical information and coaches.

2 Methods

We evaluated 5 skilled épée fencing athletes (3 female and 2 male, 20.8 ± 3.27 years, 1.76 ± 0.08 meters and 70.32 ± 10.56 kg), four of them (2 male and 2 female) were part of the Brazilian Olympic Team in 2016. After a warm-up period, each subject was instructed to perform a lunge attack from a static en garde position, at their best, while being observed by one experienced fence coach, also part of the Olympic Team.

2.1 Motion Capture and Kinematic Analysis

Three-dimensional coordinates of 39 retro-reflective markers, fixed on the lower and upper limbs, pelvis, trunk and head, were used to reconstruct whole body movements. (Figure 1).

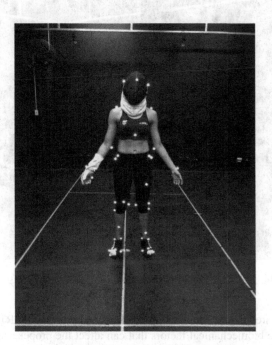

Fig. 1. Athletics with reflective marks.

Markers trajectories were captured with an OptiTrack digital motion system (Prime 13) using eighteen cameras (sampling rate: 240 Hz). The subject executed the task 5–6 times while the coach qualitatively evaluated their performance (balance and posture during lunges) according to his own criteria and corrected the gesture if necessary. Motive software (OptiTrack, version 1.8 and 1.10) was used for motion capture, reconstruction and preliminary data processing (namely, fill trajectory gap through cubic spline interpolation, in case of marker occlusion).

Data from the best-rated (BR) lunge attack of each athlete, as judged by the coach, was selected for inclusion in the 3D interactive environment, as this platform has the purpose to help in fencing trainings. Body pose during the lunge attack period was, thus, exported, for animation purposes using Biovision Hierarchy format (bvh).

Quantitative data of the following variables were made available to the coach through plots of their respective temporal series: angle relative to the anterior-posterior direction (toe in-out angle); the angle between the longitudinal axis of both feet; base length and width; horizontal position of the center of mass (CM) relative to the unarmed (back) heel; each segment, as well as the whole body, CM displacement and velocity in the forward, vertical and lateral directions; the 3D angular displacements and velocities of the upper and lower limb joints for both, armed and unarmed, sides; pelvis and trunk angular motion in the sagittal plane (Fig. 2).

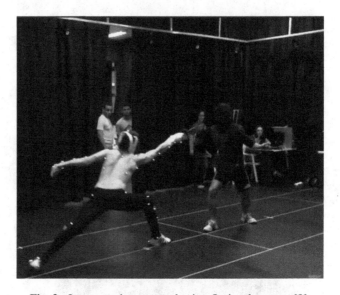

Fig. 2. Lunge motion captured using Optitrack system [9].

We also compared the kinematics of the best and worst-rated (WR) trials in order to explore further the biomechanical factors that can affect the proper accomplishment of the lunge gesture and to identify biomechanical parameters common to a group of experienced athletes that are determinant for a good lunge performance. Differently from previous studies, this approach took, primarily, into account the judgment of the individual performances established by an experienced coach.

At this step, the two best and the two worst rated trials of each athlete according to the coach criteria were used in our analysis. Calibrated Anatomical System Technique [11] was used to calculate the body segments instantaneous position and orientation. The 3D joint rotations (joint angles) were computed via Euler angles using the Cardan sequence (flexion-extension, abduction-adduction, axial rotation). Inertial characteristics of each body segment were estimated according to the Zatsiorsky-Seluyanov model modified by [12].

The calculation of the biomechanical variables selected for the performance analysis, as well as complementary data processing, were done using the Visual 3D (5.01 version, C-Motion) and Matlab software (Mathworks). The variables selected for this analysis were based on the criteria used by the coaches to judge the athlete performance [9].

2.2   Parameter Definitions to Performance Analysis

We considered attack period (T_A) to be comprised between the sudden increase of the pelvis CM velocity in the anterior-posterior direction and the instance when it drops to zero. Within T_A, the period between the front-foot ground contact loss and its subsequent return to ground (front-foot heel contact) comprises the front-leg swing phase.

We defined the period between the front-foot ground contact loss and the instance when maximum front-foot forward velocity was achieved as swing initiation (SI). For the whole T_A, we calculated: the body CM displacement and velocity; the front-foot CM displacement and velocity and the relative position of the body CM projection in the support base (CMP in base), i.e., the distance in anterior-posterior (AP) direction between the body CM projection in ground plane and the back-heel, given in percentage of the instantaneous AP distance between the back and front heel (D_{HH}). The time series were filtered using a 4th order, zero leg, low-pass Butterworth filter, with a 6 Hz cut off frequency (Fig. 3).

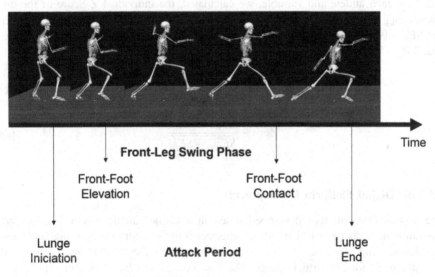

Fig. 3. Lunge parameters.

As an initial investigation, we focused on some aspects of body and front-foot kinematic. We ought to find kinematic variables that could distinguish between a well-executed and ill executed lunge. The following variables were, thus, calculated from the time series of each of the four selected trials: front-foot-step length; body CM range of motion in AP and lateral direction; vertical body CM oscillation, as well as its maximal and minimal displacement from initial position; maximal body and front-foot CM forward, downward and upward velocity; mean body and front-foot CM velocity and acceleration in AP and vertical direction, during front-leg SI; maximal high reached by the foot; maximal relative position of body CM in support base from lunge initiation to the instant front-foot lose ground contact and at front-foot heel contact and the instant maximal upward and forward velocity are reached. Displacements, velocities and accelerations were normalized by the individual's leg length and temporal variables were normalized by T_A.

Although, many statistical tools are available to identify a group of variables capable to differentiate between two conditions or groups, we choose to start from a more conservative approach. For each one of the selected variables, the mean of the two BR (m_{BR}) and the mean of the two WR trials (m_{WR}) were calculated for each athlete. In order to identify if there were biomechanical parameters that similarly affect the group performance we ran a Wilcoxon signed-rank test, for each variable, to compare the m_{BR} and the m_{WR} within the sample, adopting for that a significance level of 5%. In addition, we calculated, the mean differences between m_{BR} and m_{WR} for these athletes (m_{diff}), and the respective standard error (SE_{diff}) and, from these two quantities, the Z-score for the comparison between the group mean difference and zero mean (Z_G, Eq. 1), in order to evaluate the "size" of the difference. We also tried to identify important elements that discriminate the performance of each athlete alone. Thus, for each athlete and variable, we calculated, the individual Z-Score as the difference m_{BR} and m_{WR} divided by the standard error of this difference (Z_I, Eq. 2; SE_{WR} and SE_{BR}) [9]. We considered relevant the differences for which Z-Score were greater than 2.0.

$$Z_G = \frac{m_{diff} - 0}{SE_{diff}} \qquad (1)$$

$$Z_I = \frac{m_{WR} - m_{BR}}{\sqrt{SE_{WR}^2 - SE_{BR}^2}} \qquad (2)$$

2.3   3D Digital Platform Development

The Virtual Platform was developed based in a Game Engine. Game Engines are programming tools (mostly with visual interfaces) used in computers to make Games, Simulations and other interactive applications. Since they are currently the best available tools for 3D virtual scenes. The core system was based in Unity3D (www.unity3D.com) in addition to some add-ons such as NGUI (http://www.tasharen.com/) and others.

The system was split in modules to follow the Scrum, the adopted methodology of development. That way we could develop and integrate each module in incremental updates of the system. An eyetracking database was included in the platform as described in [13] as per coach's wishes, in order to allow future comparisons, but the results will not be discussed in this article.

The components are presented in Fig. 4.

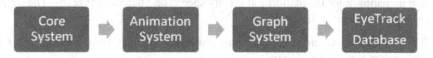

Fig. 4. System module diagram [9].

Those modules were integrated in a single stand-alone software and each function is described below:

Core System: Is the main framework where all the systems are integrated. It includes menus, 3D viewport, graphs, skeleton reconstructions and other interfaces.
Animation System: Present the captured animation using a skeleton reference where you can select bones or joints.
Graph System: Synchronized with the animations we present some graphs related to the captured movements. This includes Bone Rotation, Position and others.
Eyetrack Database: Here, the Eye Track data collected were made available.

The interface of the system was planned to be easy to use and understand, an important feature since most of the users may not have fluency in 3D interactive applications. In Fig. 5 you can see the main Mobile interface version.

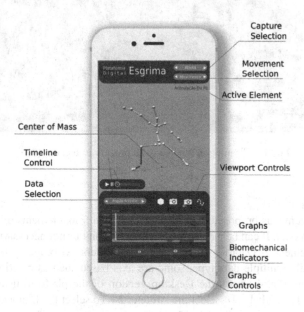

Fig. 5. Main interface of the mobile version [9].

During the development a process was implemented to insert all the data in the platform, it follows some tasks. First the model captured in BVH format was imported into Blender (www.blender.org). Blender is a Open Source 3D Software and was chosen because it allowed us to make custom scripts to import and process the animation preparing it for the platform. It greatly speeds up your work (Fig. 6). The script automates the following tasks:

1. The animations are converted to a metric scale of 0.001, that way the model gets 1:1 scale when imported in Unity.
2. All the animation poses are cleaned for wrong keyframes and the correct segment that represents the movement of interest.
3. All the segments (bones and joints) are renamed for a correct standard that we can read in the platform. It's used for the skeleton reconstruction.
4. All the data are imported and converted to a XML file. That way we can read it in the platform and plot the Graphs.

   - The model is exported as FBX format that can be read by the platform.

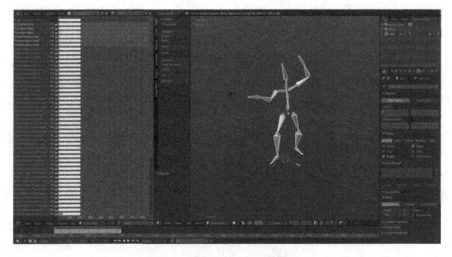

Fig. 6. Clean-up and name fixes process in blender [9].

Graph System

The Graph System was proposed to shows selected data from elements of interest from the animation model. It can be a data of a Segment, a Joint or not necessarily associated to a skeletal element as Data for gravity center and others. Also, the system is flexible enough to handle multiple data type, some are axis based such as position, others are only angles. The Fig. 4 shows the Desktop version of the platform using the Graph system (Fig. 7. Legend: 1 - To select the Athlete, 2 - To select the Element to Analyze, 3 - To select the Data, 4 - to show the Graph, 5 - To select options for instance Axis and Scale to Show).

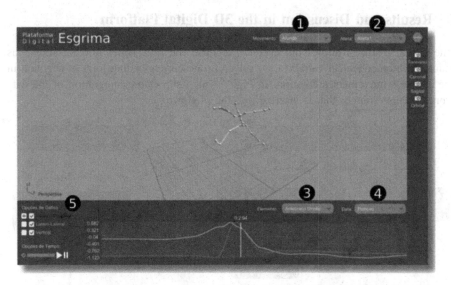

Fig. 7. Desktop platform with the graph system [9].

Eye Tracking Database

Inside the Eye Tracking Database we can find all the data collected from the eye tracking system of the athletes. The image above shows the usage of the eye tracking database (Fig. 8). It commonly contains 3 files: .tsv file with the RAW data of the Eye tracking; .xlsx file with a more accessible data that can be read in Excel; .mp4 video with the Eye tracking mirroring what the athlete sees during the execution of the movement.

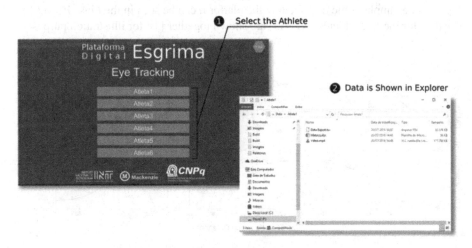

Fig. 8. Eye tracking information at the platform [9].

3 Results and Discussion in the 3D Digital Platform

The digital platform allows the user to visualize the time series and instantaneous values of biomechanical variables, by selecting the corresponding joint or segment in the athlete's movement animation. In Fig. 9 which shows the Integration of the data from different sources that is inserted into the platform.

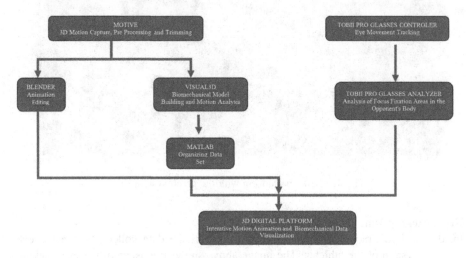

Fig. 9. Data integration into the 3D platform.

At the present, the following variables are allowed for visualization: ankle, knee, hip, wrist, elbow and shoulder joint angles at the frontal (abduction-adduction) and sagittal plane (flexion-extension), as well as the CM linear displacement and velocity for the whole body, pelvis, trunk, head, upper and lower arms, hands, feet, shanks and thighs. An example of the data feeding the platform can be seen in the Figs. 10 and 11. The data for the five athletes (A1–A5) are shown together just for illustration purposes.

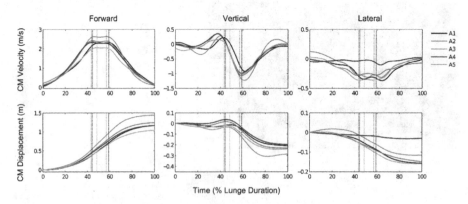

Fig. 10. Whole body center of mass (CM) displacement and velocity in the forward, vertical (upward positive) and lateral (unarmed side, positive) directions at the best performance of each one of the five athletes analyzed (A1–A5). Vertical lines indicate the instant at which CM achieved the higher forward velocity [9].

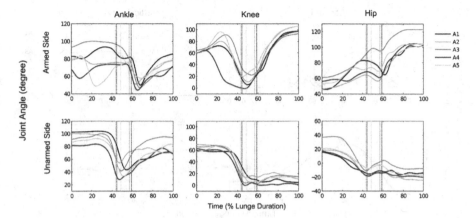

Fig. 11. Joint angle in the sagittal plane for the armed side and unarmed side lower limb joints, during a lunge attack without the presence of any target to be hit, at the best performance of each one of the five athletes analyzed (A1–A5). An increase in joint angle means joint flexion. Vertical lines indicate the instant at which the athlete's CM achieved the higher forward velocity [9].

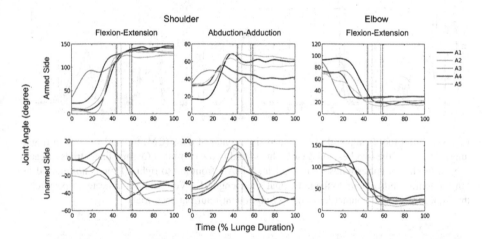

Fig. 12. Joint angle in the sagital plane (shoulder and elbow) and frontal plane (shoulder) for two of the armed side and unarmed side upper arm joints, during a lunge attack without the presence of any target to be hit, at the best performance of each one of the five athletes analyzed (A1–A5). An increase in joint angle means joint flexion and abduction, respectively. Vertical lines indicate the instant at which CM achieved the higher forward velocity [9].

3.1 Performance Results

When analyzing qualitatively the behavior of the temporal series we can notice that the athletes executed the lunge in a similar way, although synchronization between lower and upper joints (see Figs. 10 and 11), range of movement (e.g., Figs. 12 and 13) may vary considerably between them.

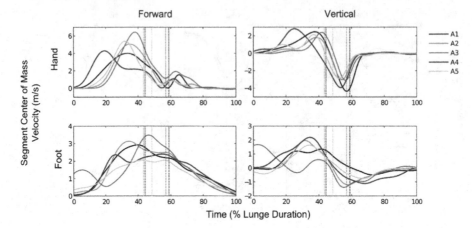

Fig. 13. Foot and hand center of mass (CM) velocity in the forward and vertical (upward positive) direction, during a lunge attack without the presence of any target to be hit, at the best performance of each one of the five athletes analyzed (A1–A5). Vertical lines indicate the instant at which CM achieved the higher forward velocity [9].

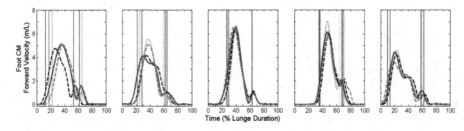

Fig. 14. Front foot (ipsilateral to the armed side) center of mass (CM) forward velocity during a lunge attack, for the two best-rated (solid lines) and two worst-rated (dashed lines) trials of each subject (each plot corresponds to one athlete; A1–A5, from left to right). Time is normalized to lunge duration and velocity to the individual's leg length (L). Vertical lines indicate, respectively, the front-foot ground contact loss and its subsequent return at each trial.

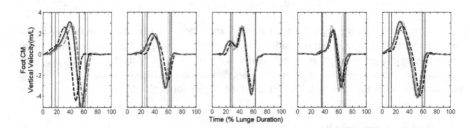

Fig. 15. Front foot (ipsilateral to the armed side) center of mass (CM) vertical velocity during a lunge attack, for the two best-rated (solid lines) and two worst-rated (dashed lines) trials of each subject (each plot corresponds to one athlete; A1–A5, from left to right). Time is normalized to lunge duration and velocity to the individual's leg length (L). Vertical lines indicate, respectively, the front-foot ground contact loss and its subsequent return at each trial.

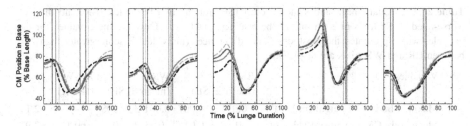

Fig. 16. Relative position of the body CM projection in the support base during a lunge attack, for the two best-rated (solid lines) and two worst-rated (dashed lines) trials of each subject (each plot corresponds to one athlete; A1–A5, from left to right). Time is normalized to lunge duration and the CM position to the instantaneous distance between both hells (base length). Vertical lines indicate, respectively, the front-foot (ipsilateral to the armed side) ground contact loss and its subsequent return at each trial.

With regard to the comparison between the BR and WR trials (respectively, solid versus dashed lines in Figs. 14, 15, and 16) it is not possible to observe a unique pattern in all the athletes differing between a well executed and a ill executed lunge. Even when comparing the four trials of the same athlete, we did not observed a well-established kinematic pattern differing the two BR and the two WR.

In addition, Wilcoxon test showed no significant differences in any of the selected variables when comparing the BR and WR trials. However, for the variables described in Table 1 the Z-score for the group exceeded the value of 2.0. When considering the athletes' performance individually, we identified relevant differences (individual Z-score greater than 2.0) in variables other than that described in Table 1 (see Table 2).

Table 1. Group mean and standard error (SE) for the variables that best distinguished the best-rated (BR) and worse-rated (WR) performances of five high-level athletes. Velocities and accelerations were normalized by leg length (L) and the relative position of body center of mass (CM) in support base is given in percentage of the instantaneous distance between heels (D_{HH}). Z-Score and the p value (Wilcoxon Test) for the comparison between BR and WR trials are also displayed.

Variables	BR (mean ± SE)	WR (mean ± SE)	BR-WR (%WR)	p	Z_G
Maximal body CM forward velocity (m s^{-1} L^{-1})	2.72 ± 0.09	2.65 ± 0.10	2.5	0.06	2.4
Mean body CM forward acceleration during front-leg SI (m s^{-2} L^{-1})	6.91 ± 0.57	6.43 ± 0.45	7.5	0.06	3.3
Front-leg stride length (m L^{-1})	1.50 ± 0.10	1.46 ± 0.10	3.0	0.12	2.6
Maximal front-foot CM forward velocity (m s^{-1} L^{-1})	5.53 ± 0.45	5.14 ± 0.45	7.5	0.06	3.4
Maximal front-foot CM downward velocity (m s^{-1} L^{-1})	3.87 ± 0.23	3.61 ± 0.23	7.3	0.06	3.2
Body CM relative position in support base (% D_{HH}) at front-foot heel contact	61.0 ± 0.9	60.4 ± 0.9	1.1	0.06	3.2

Legend: SI = swing initiation

Table 2. Individuals mean and standard error (SE) for the two best-rated (BR) and the two worse-rated (WR) trials of each one of the 5 athletes (A1–A5). Only the mean values for the variables which presented the most significant differences (individual Z score greater than 2.0) between BR and WR trials are displayed.

Sbj	Variables	BR (mean ± SE)	WR (mean ± SE)	BR-WR (%WR)	Z_I
A1	Maximal body CM height (m L^{-1})[†]	−0.021 ± 0.007	0.001 ± 0.008	–	−2.1
	Mean body CM downward velocity during front-leg SI (m s^{-2} L^{-1})	0.18 ± 0.01	0.11 ± 0.02	60.1	−2.9
	Mean body CM upward acceleration during front-leg SI (m s^{-2} L^{-1})	10.56 ± 0.79	S.77 ± 0.35	20.4	2.1
A2	Vertical oscillation range (m L^{-1})	0.025 ± 0.003	0.041 ± 0.005	−39.3	−2.7
	Instant maximal CM upward velocity is reached (%T_A)	46.8 ± 1.1	58.0 ± 1.7	−19.3	−5.5
A3	Instant front-foot heel-contact occur (%T_A)	62.5 ± 0.1	63.2 ± 0.1	−1.0	−5.5
A4	Instant maximal body CM forward velocity is reached (%T_A)	53.0 ± 0.6	56.8 ± 0.2	−6.7	−5.8
	Mean body CM forward velocity during front-leg SI (m s^{-1} L^{-1})	1.69 ± 0.01	1.35 ± 0.06	25.4	5.4
	Mean body CM downward velocity during front-leg SI (m s^{-2} L^{-1})	0.064 ± 0.054	0.251 ± 0.003	−74.5	3.4
	Mean front-foot CM forward velocity during front-leg SI (m s^{-2} L^{-1})	4.65 ± 0.31	3.84 ± 0.09	21.1	2.5
	Body CM relative position in support base (% D_{HH}) at lunge initiation	111.5 ± 4.3	99.1 ± 2.2	12.5	2.6
A5	Maximal front-foot height (m L^{-1})	0.544 ± 0.004	0.487 ± 0.004	11.5	9.4
	Maximum body CM upward velocity (m s^{-2} L^{-1})	3.12 ± 0.02	2.51 ± 077	24.4	23
	Maximum front-foot upward velocity (m s^{-2} L^{-1})	0.99 ± 0.03	0.83 ± 0.06	18.4	2.3

Legend: [†] measured from CM vertical position at lunge initiation (0%T_A): negative sign means below; SI = swing initiation.

3.2 Performance Analysis

By comparing the performance of a lunge attack in a group of five elite athletes, our results indicated that no single variable was able to be distinguish, for all the athletes, the best-rated gesture from the ones not so well performed, classified according to criteria of the coach. Such result reinforces the idea that each athlete when following the taught techniques impress in the gesture its own pattern [2, 3]. Therefore, deviations in the proper execution of this technique will have different implications in the kinematic of the movement for different subjects, and the coach when evaluating each athlete performance considered these particularities. This variability in almost all the dependent variables and the difference in time coordination was expected because the athletes have different backgrounds, different physical structures, and follow their own pattern, in spite of the usual one. These peculiarities can be a factor of performance excellence.

However the differences between the BR and WR trials, with respect to the variables shown in Table 1, seem to be relevant. Thus, coach perception of a poor performance, presumably includes lower lunge forward velocity and smaller step size, what is in accordance to [2, 8, 14].

Other subtle aspects of lunge kinematic, as the forward and downward velocities of the front-foot may also be determinant to the lunge performance independent of any particular features. We observed that front-foot maximal forward and downward velocities were 7.5% higher in the BR trials. The front-foot is accelerated not only by the forces generated by the ipsilateral knee and hip muscles but also by the energy transferred from other body segments to the front-leg. Thus, proper coordination between trunk, as well as upper and lower limb joint movement is necessary to increase front-foot velocity in both directions. Further studies should be designed to understand how energy is transferred from one segment to another in order to propel the front-foot and the body CM, as an effort to understand the effect of body segment and joint coordination on lunge performance; not only the sequential mechanical pattern of the trailing leg described by [7, 8].

Our result also indicates that the body position at front-foot heel contact can possibly be a particularly important determinant to lunge performance. We observed that even a small variation in CM position in base at this period (1.1%), resulted in relevant differences between BR and WR trials for the group. The literature [15] described that plantar pressure is higher in the front foot; [16] that fencers balance increased after training and [17] determined the foot loading characteristics of three fencing movements. None of them studied the relationship between CM position in the base and the resulting movement. This is an important variable that shows the change of weight bearing from the rear foot to the front foot and is determinant for the stability of the fencers during and after the lunge performance. This is an easy understandable variable for the coach and should be more explored.

When analyzing variables that affected individuals' performance we noticed that the relative difference between BR and WR were much higher (Table 2), which corroborate the idea that the coach may use individual criteria to judge each athlete. Vertical CM movement was indicative of poor performance for athletes A1 and A2 [1]. When A1 perform best, the body CM did not oscillate above its initial position and, during front-foot SI, the gesture was performed with a greater deceleration of body CM downward movement, while A2 oscillated in the vertical direction with a smaller range and achieved maximal upward velocity earlier in the attack period. For athlete A5, the front-leg movement was an important factor affecting performance [2]. During the BR trials, this athlete elevated the front-foot higher and with a greater velocity, what may have contributed to accelerate the body CM upward, to a greater velocity. Finally analyzing A4 performance we noticed, the body posture adopted until SI was decisive. During the BR trials, this athlete inclined further the upper body, projecting the body CM beyond the front-foot heel [2] and keeping a more unstable posture. In addition, and possibly as a consequence of the more unstable posture, during swing initiation the front-foot was moved with a greater forward velocity. In those trials, the CM was accelerated to a greater forward velocity and a lower upward swing during initiation, so that maximal CM forward velocity was achieved earlier during attack period.

These individuals analysis were important for our main interest of fulfilling the coach's needs, and give support for daily training.

4 Conclusion

The 3D platform approach is an attempt to enhance and facilitate the discussion between fencing coaches and researchers in order to explore biomechanical factors and visual aspects that may lead to an improvement on épée fencing techniques, as well as in teaching and training methods. Its support for mobile and desktop highlights the importance of visualization and interaction of the coach with results on the biomechanical parameters and visual search strategies in a more understandable and relevant way of training.

The results showed that a good lunge performance, in accordance to the coach's criteria, is very individually dependent. This great variability was expected due to the high level of the athletes. Some variables related to CM and front foot displacement seem to identify a good performance, but it is necessary for a greater sample to test this. It is not expected that a specific variable defines a good performance but that the performance suffers influence from a group of variables that interrelated. More advanced statistics will be necessary to study these possible relationships.

In general, these preliminary results are supposed to bring to light some aspects that can be responsible for a good lunge performance in fencing. But above all, this research has the aim to reassure it is necessary to establish a good relationship between the coach and the researchers, and to reinforce that we must try to find different ways of reaching the daily life of the athletes without losing the academic precision.

Acknowledgements. CNPQ is the sponsor agency of this research.

References

1. Roi, G., Bianchedi, G.: The science of fencing: implications for performance and injury prevention. Sports Med. **38**, 465–481 (2008)
2. Gholipour, M., Tabrizi, A., Farahmand, F.: Kinematics analysis of lunge fencing using stereophotogrametry. World J. Sport Sci. **1**, 32–37 (2008)
3. Chen, T.L.-W., Wong, D.W.-C., Wang, Y., Ren, S., Yan, F., Zhang, M.: Biomechanics of fencing sport: a scoping review. PLoS ONE **12**(2), e0171578 (2017). (Ed. by, T.M. Barbosa). https://doi.org/10.1371/journal.pone.0171578
4. Klauck, J., Hassan, S.E.A.: Kinematics of lower and upper extremities motions during the fencing lunge: results and training implications. In: ISBS—Conference Proceedings Archive, vol. 1, pp. 170–173 (1998)
5. Bottoms, L., Greenhalgh, A., Sinclair, J.: Kinematic determinants of weapon velocity during the fencing lunge in experienced épée fencers. Acta Bioeng. Biomech. **15**, 109–113 (2013)
6. Steward, S.L., Kopetka, B.: The kinematic determinants of speed in the fencing lunge. J. Sports Sci. **23**, 105 (2005)

7. Guilhem, G., Giroux, C., Couturier, A., Chollet, D., Rabita, G.: Mechanical and muscular coordination patterns during a high-level fencing assault. Med. Sci. Sports Exerc. **46**, 341–350 (2014)
8. Mulloy, F., Mullineaux, D., Irwin, G.: Use of the kinematic chain in the fencing attacking lunge. In: 33 International Conference on Biomechanics in Sports, Poitiers, Annals of the 33 International Conference in Biomechanics in Sports (2015)
9. Corrêa, S.C., Orselli, M.I.V., Xavier, A.P., Salles, R.J.D., Cid, L.G., Guimarães, C.P.: Kinematics fencing's analysis based on coach's criteria. In: 33 International Conference on Biomechanics in Sports, Poitiers, Annals of the 33 International Conference in Biomechanics in Sports (2015)
10. Guimaraes, C.P., Balbio, V., Cid, G.L., Zamberlan, M.C., Pastura, F., Paixao, L.: 3D virtual environment system applied to aging study - biomechanical and anthropometric approach. Proccedia Manuf. **3**, 5551–5556 (2015)
11. Capozzo, A., Catani, F., Della Croce, U., Leardini, A.: Position and orientation in space of bones during movement: anatomical frame definition and determination. Clin. Biomech. **10**, 171 (1995)
12. de Leva, P.: Adjustments to Zatsiorsky-Seluyanov's segment inertia parameters. J. Biomech. **29**(9), 1223–1230 (1996)
13. Guimarães, C.P., et al.: 3D interactive environment applied to fencing training. In: icSPORTS 2016 – Proceedings of 4th International Congress on Sport Sciences Research and Technology Support, vol. 1, pp. 05–196. SCITEPRESS - Science and Technology Publications, Lda, Porto (2016)
14. Gutierrez-Davila, M., Rojas, F.J., Antonio, R., Navarro, E.: Response timing in the lunge and target change in elite versus medium-level fencers. Eur. J. Sport Sci. **13**, 364–371 (2013)
15. Geil, M.D.: The role of footwear on kinematics and plantar foot pressure in fencing. J. Appl. Biomech. **18**, 155–162 (2002)
16. Kim, T., Kil, S., Chung, J., Moon, J., Oh, E.: Effects of specific muscle imbalance improvement training on the balance ability in elite fencers. J. Phys. Ther. Sci. **27**, 1589–1592 (2011)
17. Trautmann, C., Martinelli, N., Rosenbaum, D.: Foot loading characteristics during three fencing-specific movements. J. Sports Sci. **29**, 1585–1592 (2011). https://doi.org/10.1080/02640414.2011.605458

A Convolution Model for Prediction of Physiological Responses to Physical Exercises

Melanie Ludwig[1]([✉]), Harald G. Grohganz[2], and Alexander Asteroth[1]

[1] Hochschule Bonn-Rhein-Sieg, University o.A.S., 53757 Sankt Augustin, Germany
{melanie.ludwig,alexander.asteroth}@h-brs.de
[2] Blue Square Group e.V., 53225 Bonn, Germany
hg@blsq.org
https://www.h-brs.de/en/s4s

Abstract. An analytical convolution-based model is used to predict a person's physiological reaction to strain. Heart rate, oxygen uptake, and carbon dioxide output serve as physiological measures. Cycling ergometer tests of five male subjects are used to compare the proposed Convolution Model with a machine learning approach in form of a black box Wiener model. In these experiments, the Convolution Model yields smaller errors in prediction for all considered physiological measures. It performs very similar to other analytical models, but is based on only four parameters in its original form. A parameter reduction to one single degree of freedom is shown with comparable prediction accuracy and without significant loss of fitting accuracy.

Keywords: Prediction of physiological responses to strain ·
Heart rate prediction · $\dot{V}O_2$ prediction · $\dot{V}CO_2$ prediction

1 Introduction

Identification of the actual cardiopulmonary health status and the potential of further endurance performance is a highly relevant topic in many areas. Performance capabilities can be determined by use of different physiological measures like heart rate or respiratory gas exchange. For example, oxygen uptake ($\dot{V}O_2$) combined with heart rate can be used to determine a person's maximum oxygen uptake ($\dot{V}O_{2max}$) [11], and heart rate can be easily used to monitor the actual training or to control training intensity during treadmill exercises.

Especially heart rate is very easy to measure during exercise nowadays. If an accurate prediction (i.e., a forecast of future heart rate) shows, e.g., that a current workload will lead to an unexpected increase of the heart rate, workload can be reduced in adequate time. To ignore the limits of a person's physical capabilities will risk overtraining and will not only nullify the effect of the exercise but also reduce the subject's motivation [19,29]. Any physical mobilization and training activity for a person must therefore be highly sensitive to the person's physical

© Springer Nature Switzerland AG 2019
J. Cabri et al. (Eds.): icSPORTS 2016/2017, CCIS 975, pp. 18–35, 2019.
https://doi.org/10.1007/978-3-030-14526-2_2

capabilities and actual physical condition in order to be effective. That means that a trainer or therapist who plans the workout must be able to understand and predict with reasonable accuracy how the person's cardiovascular system will respond to a certain exercise strain, e.g., by measuring and monitoring the person's heart rate [5]. Reliable prediction can profit from models that establish a functional relationship between the strain to which the person is exposed and the response of the cardiovascular system.

Models that are suitable for individual prediction depend on a preliminary fitting process. Model specific parameters are adapted to the subject in order to fit a simulated heart rate to the measured heart rate based on a given performed strain. After fitting, the model can be used to predict a subject's heart rate for an entire training session. The planning of the training beforehand can also benefit from individualized models since personal performance limits can be considered. The process of fitting and predicting is illustrated in Fig. 1.

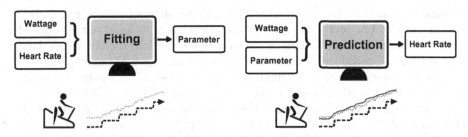

Fig. 1. Overview of fitting and prediction process. On the left-hand side, parameters of a model are fitted according to heart rate measurements and performed strain (like wattage on a cycling ergometer). With these individualized parameters, the model can then be used to predict heart rate for a different given workload before the work commences (right-hand side). The prediction can be used, e.g., to plan a training and prevent exhaustion.

These mathematical models are often based on a high number of parameters that can be rarely explained physiologically (black box or grey box models). Furthermore, a large number of parameters can lead to problems with computation time, error handling, prediction instability, and is more prone to overfitting.

In previous work [20] the authors evaluated the presented Convolution Model with regard to its general competitiveness compared to other analytical models in terms of heart rate prediction accuracy in indoor-cycling. The model proved to be the same or better in predicting the heart rate of a complete training beforehand.

On the basis of this general competitiveness, the Convolution Model is now evaluated on different types of exercise protocols. The work presented in this articel focuses on three different aspects. First, the mathematical background of the Convolution Model is examined in more detail. Second, the prediction accuracy of other physiological measures (i.e., oxygen uptake $\dot{V}O_2$, and carbon dioxide output $\dot{V}CO_2$) is analyzed as well. Third, the importance of less parameters is adressed including a more precise interpretation of the model parameters, especially in case of parameter reduction. Since the data set used in this study was originally presented by Gonzalez et al. [15] and used for prediction of heart rate and oxygen kinetics again in Gonzalez et al. [16], results from this latter study serve as a baseline for comparison.

This article begins with a brief overview of current research in modeling and predicting physical responses to strain (Sect. 2) followed by a detailed presentation of the Convolution Model and its resemblances to Hammerstein-Wiener models (Sect. 3). In Sect. 4, used data, conducted experiments, and results are presented. Discussion and interpretation of the results is given and a last section concludes the evaluation and provides some future work tasks.

2   State of the Art

A variety of models have been discussed with regard to heart rate modeling within the last ten years. Typical mathematical concepts used are systems of differential equations and Hammerstein models or variations thereof. Exemplary, Cheng et al. [8] introduce a non-linear state-space approach to model a person's heart rate behavior during treadmill walking exercises. This model was revisited by Paradiso et al. [28] and adapted to model heart rate in cycle-ergometer exercises with constant speed. In general, Hammerstein models, Wiener models, and combinations or adaptions thereof are widely used to fit physiological reactions to a certain strain, e.g., in [17,25,30,31]. One of the many variations of a Hammerstein model is a fuzzy Takagi-Sugeno model with 12 parameters by Mohammad et al. [24], which is commonly used to model physical activity of elderly untrained people. Black box models have advantages like adjusting very well to even highly varying data. For the same reason, they are very sensitive to overfitting and cannot provide any physiological insight into what's happening. Furthermore, they often need a great number of parameters to adapt to the target signal. Therefore, they are commonly used to simulate a known heart rate or predict the heart beat of the next few seconds only. The most common applications of these models are automatic control systems, particularly for treadmills or cycle ergometers. In this type of exercise, a fast system reaction is necessary for the actual heart rate, while in this case it is not necessary to simulate or predict an entire training session in advance. Usually, only some seconds up to a few minutes are predicted.

Another type of model is the linear time invariant (LTI) model by Baig et al. [2], which uses only four parameters. This model uses the latest two values of measured heart rate and strain to predict the next heart beat. It can be easily modified to predict heart rate time series of a complete physical training by estimating the heart rate iteratively and based on previously predicted heart rate values.

In an earlier study, the authors compared three different machine learning approaches and different analytical models with regard to their quality in the simulation of the heart rate and their prediction over different time horizons, as well as for the entire time series of a training (see [13,21]). In particular Linear Regression (LR), Multi-Layer Perceptron (MLP), and Support Vector Regression (SVR) were considered as machine learning approaches, and an adaption of the fuzzy Takagi-Sugeno model by Mohammad et al. [24], adaptions of differential equation models by Cheng et al. [8] and Paradiso et al. [28], and an adaption of the LTI model by Baig et al. [2]) were considered as analytical approaches. We found that machine learning approaches can accurately simulate a heart rate time series, but typically achieve similar or much poorer accuracy in predicting the heart rate of larger time horizons compared to the analytical models. Within analytical models, the fuzzy Takagi-Sugeno model achieved the best results in the simulation and prediction of a complete training time series.

Likewise, modeling of $\dot{V}O_2$ kinetics is analyzed for many years. Exemplary, Martin et al. [23] evaluated a quadratic equation used for oxygen uptake ($\dot{V}O_2$) calculation in walking within a specified walking speed range. Barnett et al. [3] presented an accelerometer calibration method to estimate the $\dot{V}O_2$ from walking after calibration on a treadmill, and Fudge et al. [12] generated $\dot{V}CO_2$ prediction equations from the combined use of acceleration measurement and heart rate in walking and running. A study on the prediction of $\dot{V}CO_2$ in treadmill walking exercises in children can be found in Morgan et al. [26]. Most of these models were derived from conducted data with regression techniques and very specific for the task of oxygen uptake modeling.

In general, the prediction of the entire time series of a body's response to strain during a training is a sparsely covered problem. A dynamic prediction model for respiratory demand during cycling exercise has been published by Gonzalez et al. [15]. In Gonzalez et al. [16], the dynamic model is extended from 10 to 12 parameters and performs accurate in simulation and prediction of $\dot{V}O_2$, $\dot{V}CO_2$, and heart rate. In the same article, Gonzalez et al. identified a Hammerstein-Wiener model as best performing black box model in order to simulate physiological measures. Further analysis in Hammerstein-Wiener models results a very good performing Wiener model as best model solution. In their analysis, the Wiener model performed better in the simulation and in the prediction of $\dot{V}O_2$, but slightly worse in terms of heart rate and $\dot{V}CO_2$ prediction compared to their extended dynamic model.

3   The Convolution Model

For the related task of predicting a measure for fitness in general, the Fitness-Fatigue model [7] has been widely used since its first description in the early seventies. It is used to calculate the actual prediction with not only the last input value but also all previous input values in decreasing intensity (exponential filter). This method means that the shorter the time between an input value and the current time, the greater the influence on the calculation of the currently calculated output value. Its great advantage is therefore a weighted consideration of the past strain with effect on the actual physiological response, performance in general or heart rate in particular. Because of the delayed reaction of human body to any strain, a model based on convolution seems to be promising to predict the heart rate response to strain. Hence, the Convolution Model is built up similarly.

Formulation of the Convolution Model can be carried out not only for heart rate but also for other physiological measures, e.g., for oxygen kinetics like $\dot{V}O_2$ and $\dot{V}CO_2$. For convenience, model description and interpretation is phrased for modeling the heart rate exemplary.

The proposed model to map the workload sequence u to a modeled heart rate sequence y was presented first in Ludwig et al. [20]. It is defined point-wise for each time t as follows:

$$y(t) = a_2 \cdot \left[\frac{1}{a_1}(u * e^{-\bullet/a_1})(t) \right]^{a_4} + a_3, \tag{1}$$

where for any functions u and x the term $(u * x)(t)$ describes the discrete convolution $\sum_\tau u(\tau) \cdot x(t - \tau)$ at time t, and $e^{-\bullet/a_1} := (\tau \mapsto e^{-\tau/a_1})$.

As earlier experiments showed [20], the four parameters allow this approach to successfully predict, e.g., a heart rate curve from a strain curve. This parametrization is not simply a mathematical trick; a physiological-phenomenological interpretation and meaning can be given to each of these parameters:

a_1 : describes the effect of former strain on the actual heart rate, i.e., how much influence previous strain has.

a_2 : explains the proportional effect of increasing strain on heart rate, i.e., it illustrates how strong the reaction to strain becomes and how steeply heart rate increases.

a_3 : a *level parameter* used as an additive constant to lift the predicted heart rate up to a suitable level. Similar to every subject's specific resting heart rate, a pre exercise heart rate can be used from which heart rate under strain ascends.

a_4 : allows a non-linear response of the heart rate to increasing strain close to the personal performance limit.

3.1   Mathematical Background

Modeling non-linear systems, e.g., for the heart rate or oxygen kinetics during exercise, is often carried out using Hammerstein-Wiener models [1,14] as pointed out in Sect. 2.

A Hammerstein model [10,18,27]—as illustrated in Fig. 2a—is used to model non-linear systems where the non-linearity is present directly at the input, so this model type consists of a non-linear function, e.g., a q-degree polynomial function

$$w(t) = f(u(t)) = a_0 + a_1 u(t) + a_2 u(t)^2 + \cdots + a_q u(t)^q, \tag{2}$$

of input signal u at time t, followed by a linear part using, e.g., a LTI model. Generally, the effect of a LTI system on some input signal is given by a convolution of the input signal with the impulse response function of the system, which characterizes the system's dynamics [9, Chap. 2.5]. So the LTI model can be illustrated by a convolution. The resulting Hammerstein model with output signal y can then be written as:

$$y(t) = (h * w)(t) = \sum_{\tau} h(\tau)w(t - \tau), \tag{3}$$

where function h is the corresponding impulse response function of the system.

Quite similar, a Wiener model [4,18]—as illustrated in Fig. 2b—is used to model non-linear systems where the non-linearity is present at the output of the system. The first part of a Wiener model therefore is a linear system which might be expressed as convolution as before,

$$w(t) = f(u(t)) = (h * u)(t) = \sum_{\tau} h(\tau)u(t - \tau), \tag{4}$$

where again function h is the corresponding impulse response function of the system, followed by the non-linear part, e.g., a q-degree polynomial function as in Eq. 2, such that the Wiener model with output signal y results in

$$y(w(t)) = a_0 + a_1 w(t) + a_2 w^2(t) + \ldots a_q w^q(t). \tag{5}$$

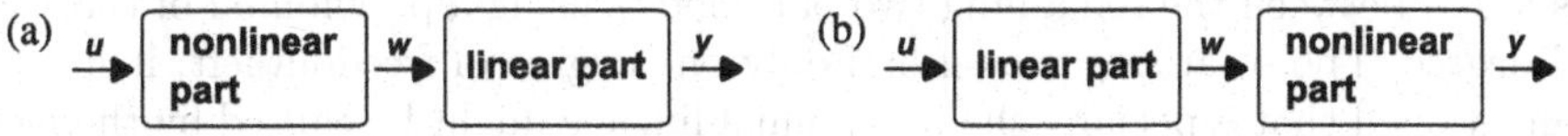

(a) $u \rightarrow$ | nonlinear part | $\xrightarrow{w}$ | linear part | $\xrightarrow{y}$ (b) $u \rightarrow$ | linear part | $\xrightarrow{w}$ | nonlinear part | $\xrightarrow{y}$

Fig. 2. Box-diagramm for (a) Hammerstein and (b) Wiener models.

Since convolution is a linear operation, we can re-formulate the Convolution Model Eq. (1) to

$$y(t) = a_2 \cdot \left[\frac{1}{a_1} \left(u * e^{-\bullet/a_1} \right)(t) \right]^{a_4} + a_3 \tag{6}$$

$$= \left[\left((\tilde{a}_2 \cdot u) * \left(\frac{1}{a_1} \cdot e^{-\bullet/a_1} \right) \right)(t) \right]^{a_4} + a_3 \tag{7}$$

$$= \left[\left(u * \left(\frac{\tilde{a}_2}{a_1} \cdot e^{-\bullet/a_1} \right) \right)(t) \right]^{a_4} + a_3, \tag{8}$$

with $\tilde{a}_2 = a_2^{1/a_4}$.

Equation 7 focuses on the role of each model parameter. Parameter $\tilde{a}_2$ scales the input u, and a_1 serves as time constant of an exponential filter. Parameters a_3 and a_4 shift and non-linearly transform the output to a suitable level. Equation 8 focuses on the usual representation of a Wiener model with the LTI part in square brackets. If we define $w(t)$ as

$$w(t) = \left(u * \left(\tfrac{\tilde{a}_2}{a_1} \cdot e^{\tfrac{\bullet}{a_1}}\right)\right)(t), \tag{9}$$

than we can define a Wiener model just following

$$y(w(t)) = (w(t))^{a_4} + a_3. \tag{10}$$

Thus, the exponential function, $\tfrac{\tilde{a}_2}{a_1} \cdot e^{\tfrac{t}{a_1}}$, is interpreted as the impulse response of the underlying LTI-system.

3.2 Parameter Reduction

Following the idea behind Occam's razor in model design (see, e.g., [22, Chapt. 28]), one aim of the Convolution Model was to find the simplest model which performs well in predicting a person's individual physiological response to strain. Especially when dealing with only a few data sets, a high number of parameters can easily lead to an overfitting and thus to inaccurate prediction results. Therefore, the number of parameters should be as small as possible without loosing accuracy.

In Ludwig et al. [20], we showed that the four parameters of the Convolution Model provide sufficient degrees of freedom and that the number of parameters might be further reduced. At first, it seems that level parameter a_3 and exponential parameter a_4 can be predefined. Additionally, a first indication of a linkage was found between the remaining two parameters using a polynomial of the second degree. The so arising model had only one degree of freedom left; it has to be mentioned that especially the polynomial linkage might be caused by the fact that all experiments of this former study followed the same step-test protocol as the same linkage cannot be found using different protocols (see Sect. 4.1). As stated before, experiments with few data sets make it indispensable to develop a stable model with few degrees of freedom.

In principle, body parameters measured while the subject is resting just before the exercise showed to be a valid additive constant for parameter a_3 to adapt the simulation to a reasonable level, but is highly dependent on the subject. The real value measured just before the training may vary depending on the form of the day but had comparatively small deviations in the analyzed data. This *individual parameter* (a_3) can be predefined for each subject based on previous training sessions.

The remaining three parameters can be interpreted as *population parameters*, depending on the general fitness of the subjects. The exponential parameter a_4 can give an idea of the physical response, especially at the beginning and at the end of a training as well as at high strain peaks. The extent of this response can decrease with higher fitness when performance reserve capacity increases during endurance training. The multiplicative parameter a_2 also strongly depends on the physical response considered, since oxygen kinetics are in completely different ranges than heart rate. Furthermore, if a person's fitness increases and a person's body adapts better to strain, oxygen can be used more effective and extent of physical reaction to strain usually decreases. Last, the parameter of the exponential filter a_1 may correlate with the multiplicative parameter a_2 as seen in our former study [20], or may even be constant as found in this analysis, Sect. 4.1.

4 Experiments

In this paper, the terms *fitting* and *prediction* are used (instead of e.g. *training* following machine learning parlance). Nevertheless, fitting describes the direct fit of parameters to given data, whereas prediction makes use of these identified parameters without any changes and applies them to different given data of the same subject. Furthermore, the term *prediction* here is meant as *session prediction*, i.e., prediction of the heart rate curve (resp. the $\dot{V}O_2$ or $\dot{V}CO_2$ curve) for a given strain over an entire training session. Especially for planning such a training session it is important to assess the physiological reaction to a given workload at a given time. While *prediction* describes the evaluation of the model on unseen training data, *simulation* describes the evaluation of the model on training data used for model fitting before. A *training* in this context always refers to physical exercise, and a *test* or *protocol test* refers to the following cycle ergometer protocol exercise tests 01–04.

Data. This dataset was originally presented by Gonzalez et al. [15]. Five healthy subjects (age: 37.8 ± 14.8 yrs; height: 180.4 ± 10.1 cm; weight: 75.2 ± 7.6 kg) completed four different cycle ergometer tests on a Cyclus2 (RBM Elektronik-Automation GmbH, Leipzig, Germany). All subjects were leisure sportsmen to well trained persons. Continuous breath-by-breath gas exchange and ventilation measurements on the mouth (Ergostik, Geratherm Respiratory GmbH, Bad Kissingen, Germany) were recorded during all tests.

The four test protocols were defined as follows (cf. Fig. 3):

1. Test 01: an incremental step test starting at a workload of 80 W with increments of 20 W every 3 min.
2. Test 02: four sprints of 6 s duration each and an incremental ramp test. Two sprints were carried out before and two after the ramp test to obtain the subject's maximal power output and $\dot{V}O_2$ profiles in a recovered and a fatigued state.
3. Test 03: a variable step protocol. The steps varied in load and duration and alternated between low and moderate or severe intensity. The linearly in- or decreasing intensity between the steps was also varied in time.
4. Test 04: a synthetic hill climb test controlled by a simulator. The gradient of that track and the subject's body weight were the major determinants of the load. While holding the same cadence as before, the subjects were able to choose their exercise intensity by gear shifting.

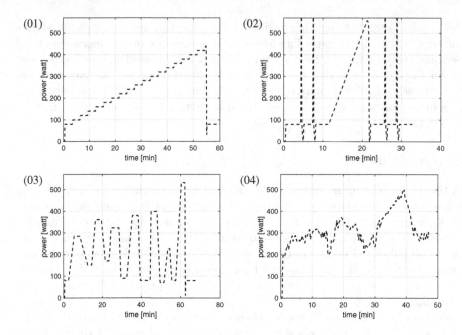

Fig. 3. Test protocols 01–04 are shown exemplary for subject #01.

In Fig. 3, the extact profiles are shown for one subject.

In [15], also smoothing and resampling were performed to reduce noise and to harmonize different sampling rates and spaces. For our experiments, we directly used the pre-processed data.

Methods. In general, heart rate models are fitted to a varying number of training sessions for one and the same person using Levenberg-Marquardt as suggested by Busso et al. [6]. The individualized model can then be used to predict further sessions.

To measure the quality and accuracy, the *root-mean-square error* (RMSE) and *mean absolute percentage error* (MAPE) are considered, where

$$\text{RMSE} = \sqrt{\frac{\sum_{t=1}^{T} (\tilde{y}(t) - y(t))^2}{T}}, \qquad \text{MAPE} = \frac{100}{T} \sum_{t=1}^{T} \left| \frac{y(t) - \tilde{y}(t)}{y(t)} \right|,$$

with T being the total number of data points, $y(t)$ the measured value at time t, and $\tilde{y}(t)$ the simulated value at time t.

The simulation was performed for each person over all executed tests, and the mean value over all persons and all tests is determined. The prediction is done in two different ways: First, the model is fitted on one single test of a person and physiological response is predicted for the remaining three tests of this person. Second, a leave-one-out cross validation is performed. We define the following prediction experiments:

1. Prediction experiment *A*: One test protocol is chosen for fitting the model, and the physiological measurements of the remaining three tests of a person are predicted. The experiments are numbered accordingly to the test used for fitting. E.g., when the model is fitted on test 01, we call the experiment *prediction experiment A.1*.
2. Prediction experiment *B*: Leave-one-out cross validation is performed. Fitting is done on three tests of a person and the remaining test is predicted. This is done for all possible combinations of the tests.

After this, the number of parameters is reduced step-by-step as reasonable as possible without loss of accuracy.

4.1 Results

Results of different experiments as described in Sect. 4 are presented below. First, simulation results are shown, followed by presentation of the prediction experiments, which yield accuracy comparable to state of the art models in all three physiological measurements. Last, the findings of the parameter reduction are presented ending in a one parameter version of the Convolution Model which yields results with comparable prediction accuracy likewise.

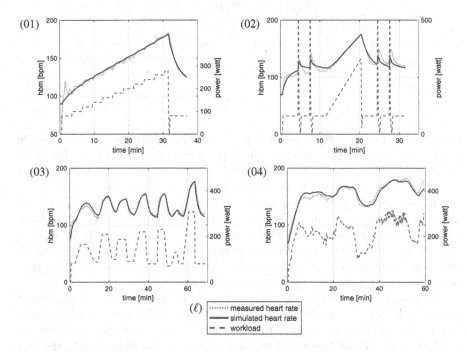

Fig. 4. Simulation of protocols 01–04 using the Convolution Model is shown exemplary for heart rate reaction of subject #05. Errors were as follows: (01) 3.69%, (02) 2.29%, (03) 2.11%, (04) 2.95%.

Simulation. First, the model was fitted for each person on all four test protocols separately. In each case, the same test as used for model fitting is simulated, i.e., reproduced. Average values over all subjects and all tests are computed. Results from Gonzalez et al. [16] are cited for comparison, and all results are illustrated in Table 1. For all considered physiological responses (heart rate and oxygen kinetics) of a person, the Wiener model proposed by Gonzalez et al. performed best. Comparing the Dynamic model and the Convolution Model, errors of the Dynamic model are less. Heart rate simulation with the Convolution Model is illustrated in Fig. 4 for one subject. In this example, test 01 has a slightly higher fitting error of 3.69% since heart rate needs some minutes to stabilize and has a short peak within the first three minutes which cannot be simulated well. The peaks from sprinting in test 02 are difficult to match as well. Simulation of test 03 yields smallest errors.

Table 1. Average RMSE and average MAPE are given for simulation of all tests over all subjects and for the three considered physiological measures. Best values are highlighted for every physiological measure.

	Heart rate		$\dot{V}O_2$		$\dot{V}CO_2$	
	RMSE	MAPE	RMSE	MAPE	RMSE	MAPE
Dynamic model [16]	4.55	2.5	0.09	3.1	0.12	4.7
Wiener model [16]	n/a	**0.9**	**0.06**	**1.8**	**0.08**	**2.9**
Convolution Model	4.95	2.92	0.13	4.0	0.18	6.60

Prediction. In the first prediction experiment, the model was fitted to a single test for each subject, and physiological responses of this subject is predicted for the three remaining tests. For the Convolution Model, resulting prediction of test 04 is shown in Fig. 5 for one subject exemplary. Results from Gonzalez et al. [16] are cited for comparison and correspond to prediction experiment $A.3$. All results are illustrated in Table 2. Comparing the Wiener model and the Convolution Model, errors of the Convolution Model are smaller for all three physiological measures within prediction experiment $A.3$. Comparing the Dynamic model and the Convolution Model, errors of the Convolution Model are higher for heart rate, and are smaller for oxygen kinetics.

Differences in prediction accuracy between different tests used for model fitting can be seen in prediction experiment A as well. Fitting on test 02 yields best results for heart rate prediction and at the same time worst results for $\dot{V}CO_2$. Comparing all different prediction setups, in case of heart rate the test choice for fitting shows no effect—variances in errors are up to 0.87%. For oxygen kinetics, errors of the prediction experiments vary around 2.24% for $\dot{V}O_2$, and around 8.6% for $\dot{V}CO_2$. The error of almost 20% in $\dot{V}CO_2$ which is achieved when the model is fitted on test 02 differs significantly[1] from results of prediction experiment $A.3$ at 5% significance level.

Table 2. Prediction of different physiological measures. Average RMSE and average MAPE are given for different types of prediction experiments (see Sect. 4) dependent on the test used for model fitting. Best values are highlighted for every physiological measure.

Experiment	Model	Heart rate		$\dot{V}O_2$		$\dot{V}CO_2$	
		RMSE	MAPE	RMSE	MAPE	RMSE	MAPE
$A.3$	Dynamic model [16]	7.46	**4.4**	0.30	8.8	0.41	12.6
	Wiener model [16]	n/a	4.8	0.27	7.5	0.44	14.2
$A.1$	Convolution Model	8.61	5.28	0.30	9.03	0.39	14.32
$A.2$	Convolution Model	7.53	4.50	**0.24**	7.66	0.49	19.96
$A.3$	Convolution Model	8.05	4.65	**0.24**	**6.79**	**0.32**	**11.36**
$A.4$	Convolution Model	8.08	5.06	0.25	7.53	0.36	12.68
B	Convolution Model	**7.34**	**4.41**	**0.24**	7.01	0.35	12.71

Prediction of heart rate is accurate for different test protocols and yields stable results independent on the data used for model fitting. Figures 6a and b show the prediction of test 01 and 02 from prediction experiment $A.3$. Figure 6c illustrates for test 04 that the prediction accuracy is independent of the data used for model fitting.

Regarding leave-one-out cross validation (prediction experiment B in Table 2), prediction errors for heart rate are smaller than those of the model fitted on only one test. This is illustrated exemplary in Fig. 6d. For respiratory measures, cross validation errors are about 0.22% higher for $\dot{V}O_2$ and about 1.35% higher for $\dot{V}CO_2$ compared to best result in experiment A.

Parameter Reduction. Since accuracy of the model is largely independent of the test used for fitting, the prediction experiment $A.3$ is used as an example for the parameter reduction. In order to stabilize the model and to reduce complexity even further, the level parameter a_3 was set to the minimal value measured before the training starts. Earlier measurements were not available. Second, the exponential parameter a_4 was analyzed between all subjects. Independently of the other remaining parameters, the exponential parameter varied around 0.6 for heart rate, around 0.75 for $\dot{V}O_2$, and around 0.8 for $\dot{V}CO_2$ and was set accordingly.

Corresponding to the steps in Ludwig et al. [20], a one parameter model can be defined again. Additionally to the predefinition of parameters a_3 and a_4 as

---

[1] MAPE values of each prediction in experiment $A.2$ are compared to MAPE values of each prediction in experiment $A.3$ with a two-sample t-test at $\alpha = 0.05$. Null hypothesis that data of both experiments comes from normal distributions with equal means and equal but unknown variances is rejected with $p < 0.01$.

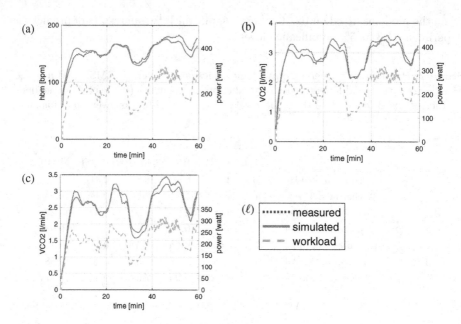

Fig. 5. Prediction of test 04 in prediction experiment A for (a) heart rate, (b) $\dot{V}O_2$, (c) $\dot{V}CO_2$ of subject #05.

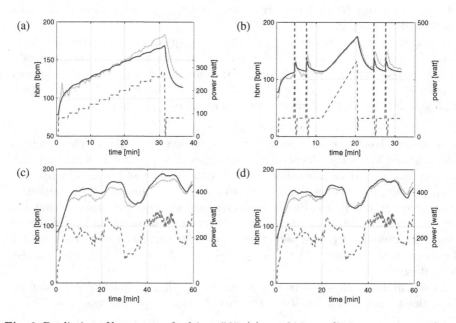

Fig. 6. Prediction of heart rate of subject #05: (a) test 01 in prediction experiment $A.3$, (b) test 02 in prediction experiment $A.3$, (c) test 04 in prediction experiment $A.1$, and (d) test 04 in prediction experiment B.

before, different possibilities for the remaining two parameters were analyzed, e.g., a polynomial linkage, a linear linkage, and a constant value for one of the two. Most stable results are reached with a constant exponential filter parameter, i.e., $a_1 = 100$ for heart rate, respectively $a_1 = 60$ for respiratory measures. The multiplicative parameter a_2 remains free. Table 3 shows results of average RMSE and MAPE for stepwise parameter reduction experiments in heart rate, $\dot{V}O_2$, and $\dot{V}CO_2$. The experiment yields comparable results for Convolution Model with one and two parameters for all three physiological measures. Even more, the one parameter model yields smaller errors than the four parameter model in the related prediction experiment $A.3$. Even if the one parameter model is used in leave-one-out cross validation, results remain comparable to the four parameter model (i.e., for heart rate: RMSE of 7.36 bpm and MAPE of 4.30%; for $\dot{V}O_2$: RMSE of 0.23 ℓ/min and MAPE of 6.94%; and for $\dot{V}CO_2$: RMSE of 0.33 ℓ/min and MAPE of 11.41%).

Table 3. Average prediction results for all three physiological measures. The model was fitted on test 03 exemplary (i.e., prediction experiment $A.3$) and the remaining tests were predicted for each subject. Before fitting, some parameters were predefined and hold in place. Results from $A.3$ of the four parameter Convolution Model are shown again for better comparison.

Predefined parameters	Heart rate		$\dot{V}O_2$		$\dot{V}CO_2$	
	RMSE	MAPE	RMSE	MAPE	RMSE	MAPE
–	8.05	4.65	0.24	6.79	0.32	11.36
a_3	8.24	4.68	0.24	7.03	0.36	12.29
a_3, a_4	8.04	4.43	0.24	7.03	0.34	10.59
a_1, a_3, a_4	7.73	4.26	0.23	6.71	0.34	10.49

4.2   Interpretation and Discussion

In order to just simulate, i.e., reproduce, a person's response to strain, the Wiener model performed most accurate with very low errors of maximum 3% for oxygen kinetics and under 1% for heart rate simulation. Since results of the Wiener model are not as good as of analytical models in prediction, the high simulation accuracy might be attributable to overfitting. Nevertheless, machine learning approaches and black box models are much more suitable when it comes to simulation. This result was already observed in former studies [13,16,21]. Prediction experiment $A.3$ shows that both analytical models, the Dynamic model from Gonzalez et al. [16] and the Convolution Model, yield highly comparable results. While the Dynamic model is more accurate in the simulation (about 0.42% for heart rate, 0.9% for $\dot{V}O_2$, and 1.9% for $\dot{V}CO_2$), the prediction results are very similar. The little higher adaptation of the Dynamic model in simulation is quite reasonable since the Dynamic model uses 12 parameter whereas the

Convolution Model gets along with only four parameters. Even more, the two parameter and one parameter versions of the Convolution Model are comparable likewise. The one parameter version performs worse in fitting, but yields slightly more accurate results in prediction as the two and the four parameter version. Following Occam's razor, reducing the model to one degree of freedom is a good and more stable choice for predicting physiological measures based on strain in cycling.

For the parameter reduction of the Convolution Model, it might be quite confusing at first view that the accuracy increases when a_3 and a_4 are predefined compared to predefinition of only a_3. This effect occurs conditioned by the test protocol used for model fitting. Exemplary for heart rate, fitting on test 03 with predefined parameter a_3 results in an average RMSE of 5.31 bpm and average MAPE of 3.31%. With predefined parameters a_3 and a_4, simulation results in an average RMSE of 5.68 bpm and average MAPE of 3.52%. While the model adapts better with fixed level parameter only and prediction of the remaining tests are worse compared to the two parameter model, the exponential parameter a_4 seems to be slightly overfitted in this case and differs more for test 03 compared to the other tests. A closer look at the exponential parameter in a comparative fitting on each test protocol separately confirms this hypothesis. Additionally, results of leave-one-out cross validation yield smaller errors for all physiological measures as results of prediction experiment $A.3$. This indicates the possibility of a light overfitting in experiment $A.3$, too. As a consequence, prediction already profits by losing one degree of freedom and predefining the exponential parameter. The higher accuracy of the one parameter Convolution Model compared to the two parameter version can be explained likewise. It has to be stated that the parameters found are dependent on the data used in this study and may change for different test protocols. In conjunction with results from our previous study [20], it seems quite reasonable that a one parameter version of the Convolution Model can be defined for different experimental settings, but the specific parameters can differ.

Overall, prediction experiment A shows that it is mostly unimportant on which data the model was fitted: predicting the heart rate was broadly independent and performed very similar for all executed test. Variances in $\dot{V}O_2$ prediction were non-significant likewise. Only prediction of $\dot{V}CO_2$ in experiment $A.2$ achieved significantly higher errors compared to results from prediction experiment $A.3$, but all other experiments again yield comparable results. So accuracy of heart rate and $\dot{V}O_2$ is mostly independent on the data used for fitting, but $\dot{V}CO_2$ sometimes causes more difficulties.

A closer look at prediction experiment B indicates that heart rate might profit most by more data used for model fitting, but prediction errors for respiration measures are quite similar than results from each best experiment and altogether better than most of the experiments in prediction experiment setting A.

5 Conclusion and Future Work

The prediction of physiological measures like heart rate, $\dot{V}O_2$, or $\dot{V}CO_2$ based on limited data can profit from a reduction of the number of free parameters in the used model. While complex models with great number of parameters can accurately fit given measurements, they tend to overfit the data, especially if data is scarce. Typically, overfitting leads to significant loss of accuracy in prediction tasks. The presented Convolution Model—a special case of a Wiener model—has in its basic form only four free parameters, an can be further restricted. Thus, the predictive accuracy can be improved. While machine learning approaches are highly suitable in terms of simulation, the Convolution Model performs better in prediction. For this task, it is as accurate as other analytical models. According to Occam's razor or the Akaike information criterion measure (AIC), the restricted Convolution Model with its fewer parametes should be chosen as a model if data is limited.

In future studies it will be necessary to verify the values that were used for fixed parameters with larger data sets. More and different test protocols as well as parameter stability will be analyzed. The model itself has the potential to be improved further. Since physiological reaction to strain is usually delayed, a constant time shift in the convolution might improve the model additionally.

An important next step will also be to analyze the usefulness of this model in simulating outdoor workouts. If training routes are known in advance, a previous simulation based on strain according to GPS profiles might be beneficial in training planning.

Furthermore, experiments using a larger data set with even more subjects trained over a longer time horizon have to prove the stability of the Convolution Model in its different versions. Particularly the one parameter version of the Convolution Model must be checked for possible overfitting. If the model remains stable, a correlation between measured changes in fitness and the remaining Convolution Model parameter can be analyzed.

Acknowledgments. The authors gratefully thank Alexander Artiga Gonzalez and the research group around Dietmar Saupe from University of Konstanz, Germany, for providing the data set used in this paper.

References

1. Bai, E.W.: An optimal two-stage identification algorithm for Hammerstein-Wiener nonlinear systems. Automatica **34**(3), 333–338 (1998)
2. Baig, D.E.Z., Su, H., Cheng, T.M., Savkin, A.V., Su, S.W., Celler, B.G.: Modeling of human heart rate response during walking, cycling and rowing. In: 2010 Annual International Conference of the IEEE Engineering in Medicine and Biology Society (EMBC), pp. 2553–2556. IEEE (2010)
3. Barnett, A., Cerin, E., Vandelanotte, C., Matsumoto, A., Jenkins, D.: Validity of treadmill-and track-based individual calibration methods for estimating free-living walking speed and VO2 using the actigraph accelerometer. BMC Sport. Sci. Med. Rehabil. **7**(1), 29 (2015)

4. Billings, S., Fakhouri, S.: Identification of nonlinear systems using the Wiener model. Electron. Lett. **13**(17), 502–504 (1977)
5. Borresen, J., Lambert, M.I.: Autonomic control of heart rate during and after exercise. Sport. Med. **38**(8), 633–646 (2008)
6. Busso, T., Denis, C., Bonnefoy, R., Geyssant, A., Lacour, J.R.: Modeling of adaptations to physical training by using a recursive least squares algorithm. J. Appl. Physiol. **82**(5), 1685–1693 (1997)
7. Calvert, T.W., Banister, E.W., Savage, M.V., Bach, T.: A systems model of the effects of training on physical performance. IEEE Trans. Syst. Man Cybern. **6**(2), 94–102 (1976)
8. Cheng, T.M., Savkin, A.V., Celler, B.G., Wang, L., Su, S.W.: A nonlinear dynamic model for heart rate response to treadmill walking exercise. In: 29th Annual International Conference of the IEEE Engineering in Medicine and Biology Society, EMBS 2007, pp. 2988–2991. IEEE (2007)
9. Chinarro, D.: System Engineering Applied to Fuenmayor Karst Aquifer (San Julián de Banzo, Huesca) and Collins Glacier (King George Island, Antarctica). ST. Springer, Cham (2014). https://doi.org/10.1007/978-3-319-08858-7
10. Eskinat, E., Johnson, S.H., Luyben, W.L.: Use of Hammerstein models in identification of nonlinear systems. AIChE J. **37**(2), 255–268 (1991)
11. Fitchett, M.: Predictability of VO2 max from submaximal cycle ergometer and bench stepping tests. Br. J. Sport. Med. **19**(2), 85–88 (1985)
12. Fudge, B.W., et al.: Estimation of oxygen uptake during fast running using accelerometry and heart rate. Med. Sci. Sport. Exerc. **39**(1), 192–198 (2007)
13. Füller, M., Meenakshi Sundaram, A., Ludwig, M., Asteroth, A., Prassler, E.: Modeling and predicting the human heart rate during running exercise. In: Helfert, M., Holzinger, A., Ziefle, M., Fred, A., O'Donoghue, J., Röcker, C. (eds.) Information and Communication Technologies for Ageing Well and e-Health. CCIS, vol. 578, pp. 106–125. Springer, Cham (2015). https://doi.org/10.1007/978-3-319-27695-3_7
14. Giri, F., Bai, E.W.: Block-Oriented Nonlinear System Identification, vol. 1. Springer, Heidelberg (2010). https://doi.org/10.1007/978-1-84996-513-2
15. Gonzalez, A.A., Bertschinger, R., Brosda, F., Dahmen, T., Thumm, P., Saupe, D.: Modeling oxygen dynamics under variable work rate. In: Proceedings of the 3rd International Congress on Sport Sciences Research and Technology Support, pp. 198–207 (2015). https://doi.org/10.5220/0005607701980207
16. Gonzalez, A.A., Bertschinger, R., Saupe, D.: Modeling VO2 and VCO2 with Hammerstein-Wiener models. In: Proceedings of the 4th International Congress on Sport Sciences Research and Technology Support (icSPORTS 2016) (2016)
17. Hadjili, M.L., Kara, K.: Modelling and control using Takagi-Sugeno fuzzy models. In: 2011 Saudi International Electronics, Communications and Photonics Conference (SIECPC), pp. 1–6. IEEE (2011)
18. Hunter, I.W., Korenberg, M.: The identification of nonlinear biological systems: Wiener and Hammerstein cascade models. Biol. Cybern. **55**(2), 135–144 (1986)
19. Lehmann, M., Foster, C., Keul, J.: Overtraining in endurance athletes: a brief review. Med. Sci. Sports Exerc. **25**(7), 854–862 (1993)
20. Ludwig, M., Grohganz, H.G., Asteroth, A.: A convolution model for heart rate prediction in physical exercise. In: Proceedings of the 4th International Congress on Sport Sciences Research and Technology Support (icSPORTS 2016), pp. 157–164 (2016)

21. Ludwig, M., Sundaram, A.M., Füller, M., Asteroth, A., Prassler, E.: On modeling the cardiovascular system and predicting the human heart rate under strain. In: Proceedings of the 1st International Conference on Information and Communication Technologies for Ageing Well and e-Health (ICT4AgingWell), pp. 106–117 (2015). https://doi.org/10.5220/0005449001060117

22. MacKay, D.J.: Information Theory, Inference and Learning Algorithms. Cambridge University Press, Cambridge (2003)

23. Martin, A., Bubb, W., Howley, E.: Predicting oxygen consumption during level walking at speeds of 80 to 130 meters per minute. Med. Sci. Sport. Exerc. **15**(2), 146 (1983)

24. Mohammad, S., Guerra, T.M., Grobois, J.M., Hecquet, B.: Heart rate control during cycling exercise using Takagi-Sugeno models. In: 18th IFAC World Congress, Milano (Italy), pp. 12783–12788 (2011)

25. Mohammad, S., Guerra, T.M., Grobois, J.M., Hecquet, B.: Heart rate modeling and robust control during cycling exercise. In: FUZZ-IEEE, pp. 1–8 (2012)

26. Morgan, D.W., et al.: Prediction of the aerobic demand of walking in children. Med. Sci. Sport. Exerc. **34**(12), 2097–2102 (2002)

27. Narendra, K., Gallman, P.: An iterative method for the identification of nonlinear systems using a Hammerstein model. IEEE Trans. Autom. Control **11**(3), 546–550 (1966)

28. Paradiso, M., Pietrosanti, S., Scalzi, S., Tomei, P., Verrelli, C.M.: Experimental heart rate regulation in cycle-ergometer exercises. IEEE Trans. Biomed. Eng. **60**(1), 135–139 (2013)

29. Smith, L.L.: Overtraining, excessive exercise, and altered immunity. Sports Med. **33**(5), 347–364 (2003)

30. Su, S.W., et al.: Optimizing heart rate regulation for safe exercise. Ann. Biomed. Eng. **38**(3), 758–768 (2010)

31. Su, S.W., Wang, L., Celler, B.G., Savkin, A.V., Guo, Y.: Identification and control for heart rate regulation during treadmill exercise. IEEE Trans. Biomed. Eng. **54**(7), 1238–1246 (2007)

Testing and Evaluation of a Differential GNSS Tracking Device for Alpine- and Cross-Country Skiing

Magnus Karlsteen[1,2], Johan Samuelsson[1,2],
and Christian Finnsgård[1,3(✉)]

[1] Centre for Sports Technology, Chalmers University of Technology,
Gothenburg, Sweden
{magnus.karlsteen, christian.finnsgard}@chalmers.se
[2] Department of Physics, Chalmers University of Technology,
Gothenburg, Sweden
[3] SSPA Sweden AB, Research, Gothenburg, Sweden

Abstract. This paper is assessing the need to find a tracking technology that can be applied in an alpine location, tracing cross country skiers as well as downhill skiers. The technology used is the differential Global Navigation Satellite System (DGNSS), a high accuracy positioning technology. The basic GNSS uses several satellite navigation systems, always providing good position coverage. The differential part adds more accuracy by using a precisely surveyed reference station. Thereby the tracked object is given a correction signals obtaining a higher accuracy on positioning data. The technology demonstrates the capability deliver accurate data, but there is a need explore the use for continuous tracking of an athlete.

Keywords: Differential GNSS · Positioning · Alpine sports · GPS · Skiing

1 Introduction

The well-known global navigation satellite system (GNSS) allows the user to measure position, velocity and local time with a highly accuracy. The global navigation satellite system's signal consists of a variety of satellite systems in space that broadcast navigation signals. The navigation signals are picked up by a GNSS receiver on the earth to determine the receiver's position and velocity. GNSS is useful in navigational applications and provides for many applications accurate enough position (2.5 m) and velocity (0.03 m/s) information. A GNSS receiver need a clear signal from at least 4 satellites to be able to deliver such data. The GNSS satellite signals are relatively weak and sometimes struggle to pass through buildings and other objects obstructing the view of the sky. GNSS can also occasionally drop out due to instabilities in the upper atmosphere. The GNSS used in this test is a differential GNSS (DGNSS). The differential GNSS uses a reference station with a precisely decided coordinate. The reference station is installed on a known position, and calculates correction parameters and sending them to and object equipped with a mobile GNSS. This method reduces

© Springer Nature Switzerland AG 2019
J. Cabri et al. (Eds.): icSPORTS 2016/2017, CCIS 975, pp. 36–54, 2019.
https://doi.org/10.1007/978-3-030-14526-2_3

the difference between the measured position and the actual true position of the GNSS user receivers [5].

The technology can be applied to several areas outside of sports. The areas of applications include for instance such as surveying, flying unmanned aerial vehicles, robotics, marine applications, and motor sports. The specifications in the project originating from a wish to apply the method for tracking of single athletes to provide exact positioning and information. As the device in this project is using differential GNSS and has support for many different satellite systems, the accuracy of the device is of interest in order to understand other possible areas of application. The intention is that the application of the technology will become wearable.

2 Problem

The problem aimed to solve is how to obtain more exact information and data on the athlete's performance to complement television broadcasts for sport events. This desired in order to give the viewer additional appreciated information by providing television companies with data services that is giving the production company an advantage over other production companies. The linking of positioning data and live video-feed is considered as extra hard to achieve. An increased precision for positioning data will provide additional features possible to combine with the viewer experience.

GNSS positioning technology can be used to obtain information on the skier's position, velocity and acceleration in both team sports and individual sports. An application for the alpine skiing environment puts demands on the positioning technology's performance and accuracy. It should also allow large capturing volumes of data to be able to analyze the run. The positioning device should not restrict in motion or cause discomfort for the tracked athlete in motion, putting demands on the size of the device.

Furthermore, the projects aim at tracking and position athletes in different contexts, providing athletes, coaches, and spectators with data. The data can be used by athletes and coaches to understand what improvements that can be made or as an escort for visually impaired athletes. The data can also be used to create a surplus value in sporting events for the spectators. The extra information that can be elicited can be used both for live spectators and for television broadcasting of sports. Extra data that can be provided to the audience is the trajectory of the slope, exact positions during the race, choice of line, velocity and acceleration [12].

A commercial differential GNSS that is comparatively low cost and small has been used. An initial evaluation and testing of the product was need, as with most surveying products, inaccuracies and errors can occur which impair the measured data.

3 Present DGNSS Research

In alpine skiing, testing and research carried out are using the differential GNSS for time measurements and force measurements. The differential GNSS that often are used in these contexts are often expensive and well calibrated and not built for applications where athletes are carrying it with them. In the research where differential GNSS are used, it is for proving the technology and accuracy of other positioning devices.

In research where athletes have carried the differential GNSS, the research performed have shown promising results in using the differential GNSS for time measurements in both alpine skiing as well as 100 m sprints. In the 100 m sprint a regular GNSS was tested and the results in the time measurements were compared to the data from a photocell. The study proves that regular GNSS can be used for time measurements of smaller segments of a slope. The technology could also be used for deciding on location comparisons between the athletes. The researchers also find data that can be used for professional athletes and their coaches to analyze training and competition performance [1]. Similar tests have been made using a differential GNSS to measure the trajectories of slopes and make time measurements with a regular GNSS to compare to the time measurements of photocells. Also in this study, tests proved that the data provided by the GNSS gives an applicable time measurement method and will provide better opportunities for analyzing the ride than from just the use of photocells for measurements [8].

Low cost GNSS using lower sampling frequencies have shown not to be appropriate for tracking and time measuring. This goes for devices using a sampling rate of 1 Hz or lower. The reason for this is the distance travelled changes too much during the sampling time [7]. The differential GNSS is also often used as a reference value when testing other positioning devices in surveying. The differential GNSS used in these cases are using real time kinematics (RTK) that provides high accuracies close to a base station. Real time kinematics uses a reference station and an open channel for broadcasts information in real time. With this information, the rover equipment is able to fix the phase ambiguities and determine its location relative to the base with high precision [2].

What can be said overall by the current research is that not many providers on the market are testing and using differential GNSS for measurements. The technology is still under development and is considered expensive and ungainly to wear in sports and is not yet considered wearable technology. The present research involves testing and concept proofing along with software development that is leading to the finished product. Much of the effort going down in the project have been accuracy between two or more units. Before the tests performed in this project no calibrated testing had been made.

The testing performed gave numbers on exactness among the devices. Previously tests applying the technology on racehorses had been carried out. The initial idea with the technology was to be able to track the horses on harness races. The intention was to provide television broadcasting extra value in the form of horse tracking. To demonstrate the tracking technology, graphical representations as well as some accuracy calculations was used. The evaluation method used when initiating the project was made by using graphical evaluations of the accuracy. The graphical evaluation had been developed by calculating a graphical coefficient using a satellite photo of the current position to get a value using the latitude and longitude measurements. This called for calculations of the coefficient for each location that the tests were performed on.

From the above background and described problems, the purpose of this paper is to evaluate a differential GNSS tracking technology and whether it can be applied in alpine- and cross-country skiing.

4 Theory

Satellite based positioning is the determination of positions of observing sites. Satellites provide the user with the capability of determining a position expressed by for instance latitude, longitude and height.

Latitude and longitude can be described as the angle between where the object is positioned and the reference axis. For latitude, the reference axis is the equator. For longitude, the reference meridian is the international prime meridian. This way, every location on earth can be specified by a set of numbers. Latitude is specified as the lateral positions on a spherical shape, and the longitude as the vertical positions on a spherical shape. The latitude and longitude is measured in degrees or radians. The altitude that needs to be used when specifying positions is measured in meters over the reference ellipsoid WGS84, a model used for approximating sea level across the Earth [3].

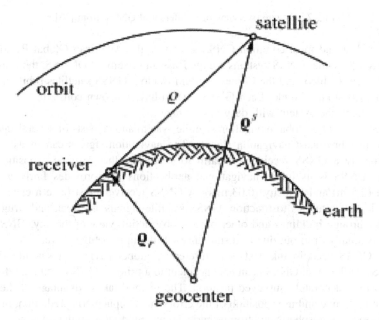

Fig. 1. Principle of satellite based positioning [3].

The process for positioning something with latitude, longitude and elevation is done by a resection process, where range differences measured to satellites are used, see Fig. 1. To relate this to what is happening, the vector Qs relates to the center of the earth (geocenter) of each satellite. The geocentric position of the receiver on the ground is defined by the vector Qr and is set to system time. The geometric distance Q to each satellite could be measured from recording the time required for the satellite signal to reach the receiver. Using this technique would yield in the unknowns, latitude, longitude, and elevation, that could be determined from the three range equations $Q = \|Qs - Qr\|$ [3].

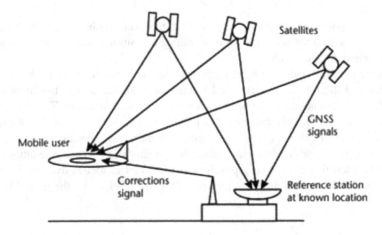

Fig. 2. System overview of a differential GNSS, from [13].

The oldest and most common GNSS system is the American Global Positioning System (GPS). Other GNSS systems are the Russian system GLONASS, the European Union system Galileo, and the Chinese system Beidou. GNSS satellites orbit the earth at about 20,000 km altitude. Each GNSS system has their own constellation of satellites, providing the system with desired coverage.

GNSS stands for global navigation satellite system and consists of several satellites in space that broadcast navigation signals. The navigation signals can in its turn be picked up by a GNSS receiver on earth to determine that receiver's position and velocity. GNSS is useful in navigational applications and provides fairly accurate position (2.5 m) and velocity (0.03 m/s). A GNSS receiver must have a clear signal from at least 4 satellites to function. GNSS satellite signals are weak and struggle to penetrate through buildings and other objects obstructing view of the sky. GNSS can also occasionally drop out due to disturbances in the upper atmosphere.

The GNSS used in this test is a differential global navigation satellite system (DGNSS). Differential GNSS is an enhancement to a primary GNSS, using a reference station with a accurately surveyed position. The method takes advantage of the slow variation with time and user position of the errors due to ephemeris prediction, residual satellite clocks, ionospheric and tropospheric delays. Starting from the reference station the system broadcasts corrections to the GNSS rover, see Fig. 2. The rover needs to be enabled for receiving correction signals and be connected to the same satellite as the reference station in order to function [3, 4].

This technology results in a reduction of the deviation of the measured position to the actual position of the GNSS user receivers. The reference station has the technical possibility to position itself using different satellite systems, which leads to a more accurate position. Variations of the technology exist, where multiple reference stations are used, leading to a higher accuracy for the rover. This technology can be applied to cover a larger area, using reference stations strategically placed to have coverage on the correction signals.

When processing the data coming from the units, the error and standard deviation needs to be expressed in an easy comparable unit. The unit of choice was meters, to get a physical translation that is relatable. This yields for transformations of the data. According to Advanced Navigation, their procedure was to do the transformation to Earth Centered Earth Fixed (ECEF) [10].

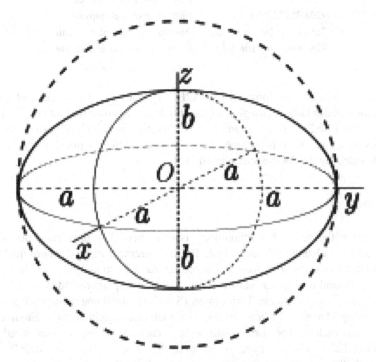

Fig. 3. A sphere of radius a compressed into ellipsoid, from [13].

This format is useful in calculation of Cartesian coordinates when using a non-spherical form. Converting in to Cartesian coordinates and considers the earth as a sphere will yield in a systematic error in the measurements, as the earth is not spherical, see Fig. 3. This means that if calculating with Cartesian coordinates and using the same radius for the entire earth would yield in different errors at different locations. Using ECEF conversion the earth is considered an elliptical shape and the flattening of the earth will be considered in the calculations. The Cartesian coordinates calculated will have its origin in the center of the earth. The geodetic coordinates will be transformed from latitude and longitude into X and Y coordinates while the altitude will be added to the Z-component to get the altitude and the change thereof. The altitude of the Z-component will be expressed in meters above the reference ellipsoid.

World Geodetic System 1984 (WGS84) is a terrestrial reference frame, a reference ellipsoid. The reference ellipsoid is a mathematically defined way of describing the surface of a geoid. Associated with this frame is a geocentric ellipsoid of revolution, originally defined by the parameters a, f, ωe and μ, see Table 1. WGS84 is globally considered accurate within 1 m [3].

Table 1. Parameters of the WGS-84 ellipsoid [13].

Parameter and value	Description
a = 6378137.0 m	Semimajor axis of the ellipsoid
f = 1/298.257223563	Flattening of the ellipsoid
!e = 7292115 · 10 − 11 rad/s^{-1}	Angular velocity of the earth
μ = 3986004.418 · 108 m^3 s^{-2}	Earth's gravitational constant

Using the Matlab [6] command LLA2ECEF from the aerospace toolbox, the geodetic coordinates latitude, longitude and altitude where converted into ECEF-format in meters. The LLA2ECEF command is using WGS84 as default ellipsoid. The input arguments for LLA2ECEF is [degree, degree, meters], which is fitting for the data set that is provided by the DGNSS examined [11].

5 Method

In this section the research methodology is described. The data collection design together with data handling is described. The measurement method where made with accurately surveyed positions were calibrated on flat ground and in a ski slope.

The flat ground testing was performed on Vallhamra sports facilities (Sweden) and the ski slope of choice was in Ulricehamn (Sweden). By doing post-processing calculations using Matlab and Microsoft Excel, the latitude, longitude and altitude can be translated into meters. The used points were accurately surveyed using hired technology from Leica. The surveyed points were then put on the form fitted for comparison with the data points from the tested product. By hiring the technology, a reference value could be established, and thereby minimize sources of errors in reference. By putting the GNSS antenna in the zigzag pattern and allowing it to collect 180 samples the point is considered accurately surveyed and the position is known with 3 mm + 0.1 ppm accuracy.

The tests carried out on Vallhamra sports facilities where replicated in a slope at Ulricehamn ski center. The proceed was the same using hired technology from Leica to survey points in the slope, marking out these and thereafter make a run on skis, wearing the devices mounted on top of the helmet. When processing the data coming from the units, the error and standard deviation needs to be expressed Physical testing have been performed on flat ground and in a slope. The flat ground tests were performed for getting a value where accuracy could be calculated. This accuracy was then applied on the tests in the ski slope as a proof of concept. The tests were made with regard to finding absolute accuracy and the relative accuracy. To get a value of the absolute accuracy, accurately surveyed points on a plane surface is being marked out using a levelled Leica Viva GNSS GS14 together with a hand-held Leica CS20, see Fig. 4.

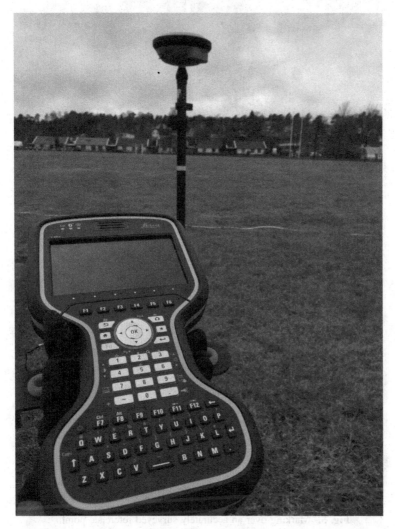

Fig. 4. Surveying of positions using Leica GS14 GNSS antenna and a handheld Leica CS20 controller.

Here the exact position can be compared to the value from the GNSS unit. The accurately surveyed points on the sport arena were placed in a zigzag pattern. The points were marked using orange spray paint and thereafter visited one at a time. By holding the GNSS over the point for five seconds, a visual trigger was provided for the post-processing of data, providing the possibility to see where the points are, as seen in Fig. 5.

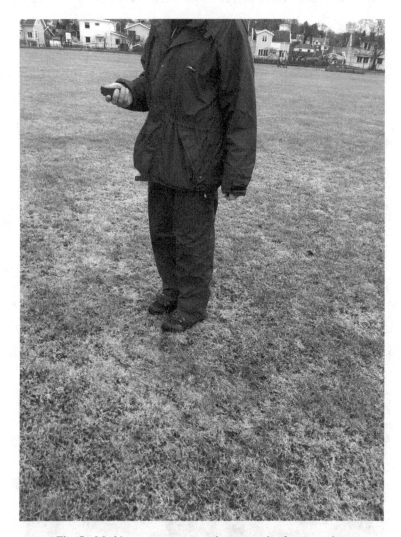

Fig. 5. Marking over an accurately surveyed reference point.

Both the flat ground tests and the tests performed in a ski slope were made using a calibrated starting point and then 4 other points in a zigzag pattern. The points are calibrated with the Leica Viva GNSS GS14 mounted in the point, using averaging for

160 cycles, and thereafter marked out, using an orange spray paint. The collection of data was made after calibrating points. After this the devices where hand held and walked across the field. At each point the device was held still for five seconds to mark the position in data. This yielded, with a sample rate of 20 Hz, 100 samples at the position, making it possible to read out from the data sheet. By plotting the data, an estimation of at what sample the position is marked. This sample number is then translated from its (latitude, longitude, altitude)-form to an earth centered, earth fixed, ECEF-form. This will yield in a format of the coordinates and the movement can be given in a form of a regular coordinate system (X, Y, Z). The movement given in ECEF-form will then be used for creating a mean value around the turning point. The mean value is calculated around the minimal difference value using 90 samples. From these values a standard deviation and mean error for the accuracy was calculated.

Investigating the accuracy between two devices was made by putting two or more units on a fix distance between the units. Here the recorded distance can be compared to the actual distance. This testing was only performed on flat ground. The testing was performed using a plank attached to a bicycle holder in the back of a car. This car was then driven around a running track. The two units attached to the plank were then observed and the distance between them, 188 cm, could be observed how it differed from the reality. From this data the standard deviation and mean error can be calculated. The recording of the distance between the devices is made by using a plugin for the program recording the data. Gmap.net and mapprovider.projection.getDistance are the plugins and functions that are used by the program.

6 Results

For the flat ground test with calibrated points the test was made using two different trackers. The data was processed separately from that data set and thereafter analyzed. The accurately surveyed latitude and longitude will be denoted CALLAT and

Table 2. ECEF values for tracker 2 at Vallhamra [m] [13].

ECEF		
callat	callon	calalt
3,33842098697508	7,14501958786384	5,36952170358413
3,33844662508295	7,14486992245528	5,36950821375262
3,33842131184515	7,14446474910573	5,36952914614575
3,33845256235963	7,14444444701532	5,36951029111727
3,33844085223223	7,14414386226753	5,36952130994464
deltalat	deltalon	deltaalt
3,33842141172043	7,14502271428875	5,36952240952373
3,33844698028778	7,14486932115255	5,36950865646570
3,33842142120938	7,14446502922780	5,36952956020196
3,33845203372697	7,14444354158593	5,36950945065900
3,33844040391479	7,14414568630733	5,36952059257905

CALLON. The values used around the turning points when doing the tests are denoted lat and the mean value around that point is denoted Δ*lat* and Δ*lon*.

The columns ECEF means that the values have been converted from lat, lon, alt into earth-centered earth-fixed, ECEF-form. This was done using Matlab and converts an input of ([rad], [rad], [m]) into ([m], [m], [m]). The Matlab code uses the following values for WGS84 ellipsoid constants [9]. The final column Diff is simply the difference between the calibrated value and the mean value around the turning point. This is the same as the distance from the calibrated point (Table 2).

For tracker 2 the RMS values for the different positions were 0.5274, 0.36026, 0.11289, 0.53633, and 0.484 m for each point. This results in a standard deviation of 0.1773 m. For tracker 3 the RMS values for the different positions were 0.0768, 0.3877, 0.5563, 0.9203, and 0.4331 m for each point. This results in a standard deviation of 0.3053 m.

Tests on relative positioning error was also made by putting two devices on a fix distance between them and then driven around a running track with a car. The physical distance between the devices was 1880 mm and in Fig. 6 the fluctuations in difference can be seen over the 2200 samples. The setup is shown in Fig. 7. The calculations from this gives a standard deviation of 1.003 m, a mean value of 0.215 mm and fluctuating values between −1.877 m and 2.321 m.

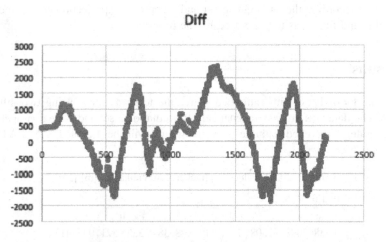

Fig. 6. Positioning error, distance [mm] between two units over sample number [n] [13].

This means that mean of the two trackers results in a standard deviation of 0.2413 m (Table 3). So, with 68% certainty the data retrieved from the tracking device is within a span of 0.2413 m of the observed position. With 95% certainty the data from the tracking device the device is within a span of 0.4826 m of the observed position. With 99.7% certainty the data from the tracking device the device is within a span of 0.7239 m of the observed position.

Physical testing in the intended environment of use was also made. This was made as a proof of concept, that the device can be used for tracking an alpine skier. In Figs. 8

Table 3. Standard deviation of the measurements from Vallhamra IP [13].

1$\ddagger$	2$\ddagger$	3$\ddagger$
64%	95%	99.7%
0.2453 m	0.4426 m	0.7239 m

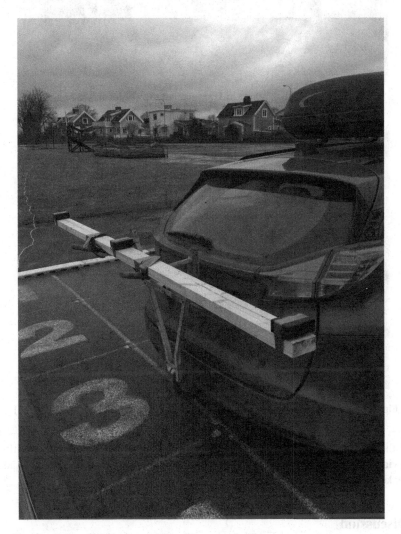

Fig. 7. Setup of devices on Vallharma sports facilities to test relative accuracy.

and 9, a red and a blue line can be observed. These lines are both representing a rover carried by a skier. The red line is following the track that was surveyed. The blue line is another of the rover, that drifted away and did not provide any results of use. When

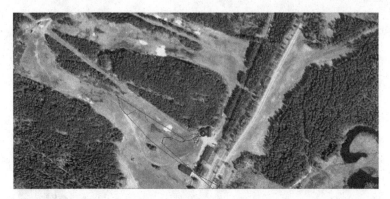

Fig. 8. Run from ski slope in Ulricehamn [13]. (Color figure online)

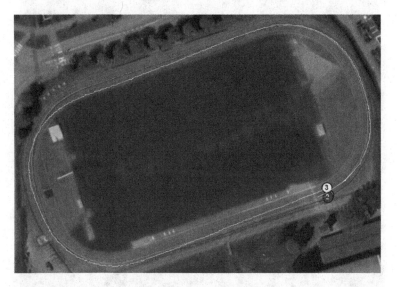

Fig. 9. Measurements from Vallhamra sports facilities [13]. (Color figure online)

riding the lift for the ski slope test, the connection was lost when going up the lift and the devices needed to be restarted. After this, the data collection could proceed and in the peaks, the turns can be observed.

7 Discussion

After some research on methods of how to translate the data available, it was decided to take the approach using accurately surveyed points. Holding the rovers laying flat in the palm of the hand, the accurately surveyed points were marked one at a time by holding the rover still for five seconds. Mean error and standard deviation was than calculated by taking the difference between this point and the points close to the point. This could yield in a better accuracy than reality, since the data collection was allowed to run while being close to the point. When calculating the mean error in this case, the measurement is assumed to reach a steady state with close to zero error. Therefore the outcome from these results should be approached with caution as they might leave a too promising prognosis.

The accuracy from the tests was better than expected. As earlier stated, the accuracy should be approached with caution, as the method is not verified. It is hard to further discuss whether the accuracy is good enough or not, regarding what requirements and future areas of use into a value to aim for.

After performing the tests it was found that the calibration of altitude should have been made before commencing the collection of data but was not made properly which resulted in a systematic error of 5.4 m. This calibration is made with regard to the height above the ground that the reference station is put. This was handled when doing the post processing of the data. The calculations were performed with the systematic error subtracted in order to not affect the data. The subtraction was made in order to get a proper value of the altitude measurements, as these are important when measuring in a ski slope.

The values on the relative positioning error was not as good as expected. Earlier measurements performed by a company had shown more promising results. The reason for this could be that there have been a problem with getting a differential fix between the reference station and the devices, something that was experienced during the tests. Earlier tests have shown standard deviations and mean errors that were more in the range of 0.7 m and 0.003 m in mean error according to the company contact. This method of testing should however be considered to be discarded. To calculate the error between two unsure sources should not be considered as a scientific way of proving performance for a product like this. The way errors occur for two rovers among them can be random and if interference of the satellite signal occurs, it will do so for both of them, causing unreliable results.

It is important outcome from the testing in the ski slope, is that when connection is lost for the device it is crucial to restart it and allow it to get a differential fix before commencing the tests. Reasons for the blue line in Fig. 8 can be because of this problem. The rover has failed to get differential fix and the collected data is useless. The problem can also have appeared because of problems with the software causing multi-path errors. After the study, a software update has been performed, targeting a number of weaknesses. A follow up study showed considerably better results.

Alternative methods for measuring are present. The most used method is continuous measurements using a calibrated differential GNSS. Post measurements data processing then needs to be made using Matlab or software such as Justin from Javad, where one can evaluate data from two different input sources in double differential mode. In a comparison of cost between choosing to go with Matlab versus investing in Justin it differs 2800 SEK between getting Justin from Javad. Matlab 18500 SEK + aerospace toolbox 9500 SEK = 28000 SEK versus Justin from Javad 30800 SEK. [6].

The method using accurately surveyed points put demands on post processing data handling that was time consuming. The time consumption is not in parity with the power of the results, as the method is not verified when evaluating GNSS accuracies.

This is another reason for investing in software for facilitate quick evaluations of future updates in the product.

The tests showed that the units where non-robust to rotation, something that caused the unit to lose the differential fix. This needs to be evaluated in a future requirement specification whether it will be a problem when using.

8 Conclusion

Wearable tech is an expanding market and the rate of emerging companies is high. Many different products and technologies exist on the market. Ranging from GPS watches to ungainly differential GNSS, the competition is extensive. A differential, wearable GNSS with stable data collection would generate a new area for tracking and positioning devices. The wearable technology, using differential GNSS with an accuracy that could pose a threat to this product ha focused their development effort towards virtual reality products. It should be kept in mind that this kind of technology is growing in many different areas of technology and are widely spread. By specifying what the product is going to be used for, whether it is time measurement, line choice of the skiers or measurements of velocity, etcetera.

The recommendation when pursuing the market of differential GNSS tracking of athletes, is to standardize the testing method. Since the product has not yet reached its final technology and the implementation of real time kinematics, it should be considered favorable to have a standardized method for testing where improvements can be confirmed. The standardized method needs to be created to be able to process data in a reasonable way where improvements can be easily recorded.

The next step when reaching a prototype that is reaching the requirements for the product and testing in different environments and possible sources of error and most favorable conditions for testing. The technical possibility for switching between antennas is already implemented but not yet evaluated and should therefor also be evaluated. This will be vital to provide signal range for a full ski slope or a cross-country ski slope.

At present there are several factors with the devices that are not making it robust enough for use. Tilting of the devices, calibration of height over the ground and loss of differential fix when put in a skip zone are all problems that is pointing towards an unfinished product. These findings should be put in the requirements specification if they pose a threat to a functioning problem. The earlier these problems can be resolved, the cheaper it can be fixed rather than having to do late changes in product development process.

As the product is acquired from a company, the technical knowledge is coming from this company to a large extent. All the hardware updates will be manufactured and updated by professionals as soon as the technology is available. This company is also providing software updates when needed. The company also provided technical support, both remote and by doing hardware updates when needed. This makes the down time for a non-functioning product low, which is desirable when trying to develop a product and keeping the time to market low. It should also be considered a asset that the implementation of both differential GNSS and RTK is not wide spread on the market of sports tracking. Harvesting the technology and being first on the market is favorable, especially when having potential customers and users wanting to be a part of the requirements specification. This will help the development process towards reaching and putting out a finalized product.

The current technology is limited in credibility as random numbers and systematic errors occur. This calls for ongoing quality checkups to ensure that the data collected is in order. The test data needs to go through extensive post testing processing to be able to study possible sources of error. By developing a test method, this time could be reduced and improvements can more easily be recorded. This will in its turn faster provide feedback and the possibility to reach out to possible customers, presenting their technology. The current version lacks a possibility for data recording, only live tracking is possible. The transmission of data resolution of live tracking is high in the current version is not as high as the hardware permits. The transmission rate is what limits the current version of the device.

The products could be updated to be able to record data in future prototypes if this is considered to be of importance. As the product is going to go through hardware updates, implementing real time kinematics (RTK) during 2017, other hardware updates are still possible. The battery time of the devices needs to be evaluated. As the devices are updated, the battery time might change. The slimmer and more lightweight a device needs to be, the slimmer the battery will need to be. Coupling this with power-intensive analysis tasks such as position and tracking, the performance can suffer. It is also possible to change settings on what to measure. As the devices have various different sensors, the energy consumption on these needs to be taken in account. Making sure that what is measured is made use of is a way of saving energy for what is necessary for the tests and in its applications.

The competition in differential GNSS trackers that are ruggedized and fit for using in sports tracking is limited. The technical opportunities are many in terms of being first on the market in tracking with this accuracy. By taking advantage of the cooperation with the producing company the technical development and hardships occurring can more easily be resolved and the time to market can be kept short. Doing this, it will be crucial to keep good business relations with the producing company. The company has a good opportunity to be the first on the market in differential GNSS. The accuracy that will come with implementing RTK will make them head of sports tracking if being able to finalize a product and make it reach the market in low development time.

The positioning of the reference station is vital for acquiring optimal signal when transceiving to a GNSS rover. The reference station itself can experience trouble in getting coverage. Factors such as the weather and vicinity to water or other reflective surfaces might cause signal disturbance. Since water and reflective surfaces previously have caused trouble in the path of the rovers, investigation on performance on ice needs to be done as the slopes in ski racing often are prepared to be icy. The implementation of Real Time Kinematics (RTK) is a prospect development that is going to be made by the Technology Provider. This implementation itself might lead to problems arising, which needs to be taken in account in the development process. For covering larger areas of tracks in for instance cross country skiing, the differential GNSS will need to be able to shift from one antenna to another. This functionality is according to the Technology Provider already implemented. However, the technology needs to be evaluated in the environment to ensure accuracy and flawless transitions between antennas.

The project needs to specify what accuracy is wanted in order to deploy the technology. Putting together a requirements list will help in deciding when to stop the development, when the accuracy is sufficient. Making a requirements list for both the virtual escort as well as the tracker for alpine sports will give a indication on the development effort that have to be put in the project. This can also indicate whether differential GNSS is a good investment or if an accurate regular GNSS device will be sufficient. It will also indicate whether investment in implementing RTK is necessary. The project currently lacks a fast way of evaluating the technology, or seeing how improvements are made. A general recommendation for faster evaluations on technical software and hardware updates is to acquire a technique or a software to make swifter evaluations on the changes.

The project will enter new phases where the technology is going to be used in different ways. By establishing a wanted accuracy in these different projects will make it possible to realize when the development is ready to be taken into the next phase. To strive for good accuracy without an aim will make it possible to never stop try to improve the accuracy. To ensure an early market introduction, it will be crucial to get the technology sufficient for the intended purpose and thereafter move on.

If one of the intended areas of use shows to have a higher demand on the accuracy, the development of the product can be made in parallel, cutting development time. Therefor it should be considered crucial to make the requirements specification for both of the separate parts of the project. In all development projects it is important to translate demands and wishes on a finalized product into a requirements specification made up of numbers or factors that can be measured and verified. By getting a number on how accurate the technology needs to be, it will be tangible when the development of the positioning technology is finished. This requirements specification will also provide the development project with a physical representation of what the accuracy will mean practically.

An investment in a software for evaluations of accuracy. Dedicated softwares for this can provide a fast evaluation. The Technology Provider are using Matlab, but a more reasonable investment to do in this case is probably to use a dedicated software for GNSS evaluation. Justin Javad, RTKLIB, GPSTk, trackRT, Bernese and Trimble are all examples of softwares that can be used to evaluate accuracy of GNSS devices. Among them are several open source softwares, as well as license software that can be used for this application.

This consideration needs to be made on a basis of what software proficiency that is available in the company. If choosing Matlab, development costs will follow with the investment. On the other hand, using an open source software might put demands on further software development. These numbers are just put as an example for the company to choose side. The main focus from the company is to have someone who have knowledge in the technology they choose.

In order to maintain the technical advantage, the company should consider making the investments in updating their technology to Real Time Kinematics. As many of the competitors have tracking possibilities with varying accuracies, it should be considered a profitable investment to be first in the area of sports tracking using differential GNSS with RTK, improving the accuracy and creating a product that currently lacks competition on the market.

When performing future accuracy evaluations, a reference track should be used in order to continuously evaluate updates. By having a consistency in the evaluation method, the evaluation gets more reliable. The creation of the reference track should be made simultaneously with the data collection of the differential GNSS. There are two reasons for this, to be able to synchronize the data sets and to ensure that the circumstances of the earth is the same for the two different data sets.

When performing tests, it is important to make everything at the largest extent possible, replicable. Therefore, it is suggested to use the same algorithm for the process every time. In the next section a specified algorithm will be presented. Other factors that might affect the measurements that should be considered when collecting data are the following

- Collect data in clear weather in order to ensure satellite coverage. Cloudy skies might prohibit signal coverage.
- Collection of data to be analyzed should be made continuously, instead of around accurately surveyed points.
- The rovers need to be restarted and get differential fix before commencing data collection.
- The rovers must be carried with the right side up, and with the correct side in front. The rovers should not be rotated over 40° in order to not loose contact with the reference station.
- The reference station needs to be calibrated in height over ground every time when performing tests. This is important to remember, otherwise it will result in a systematic error in the altitude measurements, something that is important to do as accurate as possible when tracking alpine skiers.

Acknowledgements. The authors wish to acknowledge the support from Chalmers Area of Advance Materials Science, and the Department of Physics of University of Gothenburg. And Västra Götalandsregionen via Regionutvecklingsnämnden for its financial support Finally the support from New Century Information AB, with Bengt Julin, Anders Yttergård and Klas Öberg is highly appreciated.

References

1. Advanced Navigation: Spatial (2015). http://www.advancednavigation.com.au/product/spatial#applications. Accessed 26 May 2016
2. Advanced Navigation: Spatial (2016). http://www.advancednavigation.com.au/product/spatial#documentation. Accessed 30 May 2016
3. Hofmann-Wellenhof, B., Lichtenegger, H., Wasle, E.: GNSS – Global Navigation Satellite Systems. Springer, Wien (2008). https://doi.org/10.1007/978-3-211-73017-1
4. GMV: DGNSS Fundamentals (2011). http://www.navipedia.net/index.php/DGNSS_Fundamentals. Accessed 12 May 2016
5. Granby, P.: Unpublished M.Sc. thesis, Chalmers University of Technology Javad. Justin (2016). http://www.javad.com/jgnss/products/software/justin.html#. Accessed 05 June 2016

6. Matlab: Pricing and Licensing Aerospace Toolbox (2016). http://se.mathworks.com/pricing-licensing/index.html?prodcode=AT&s_iid=main_pl_AT_tb. Accessed 05 June 2016
7. Mercator, P.: Leica Viva GS14 – GNSS Smart Antenna (2016). http://leica-geosystems.com/products/gnss-systems/smart-antennas/leica-viva-gs14. Accessed 16 May 2016
8. Murray, S.: Putting Wearables into Context with Low-Power GNSS (2014). http://www.broadcom.com/blog/wireless-technology/putting-wearables-into-context-with-low-power-gnss/. Accessed 09 May 2016
9. National Imagery and Mapping Agency: World geodetic system 1984. Technical report NIMA TR8350.2, Department of Defense (2004)
10. Orr. X.: NCI sports tracker project - the road ahead... Unpublished Company Material (2016)
11. Statista: Big Data Market Size Revenue Forecast Worldwide from 2011 to 2026 (in billion U.S. dollars) (2016). http://www.statista.com/statistics/254266/global-big-data-market-forecast/. Accessed 29 Feb 2016
12. Spörri, J., Limpach, P., Geiger, A., Gilgien, M., Müller, E.: The effect of different global navigation satellite system methods on positioning accuracy in elite alpine skiing. Sensors **14** (10), 18433–18453 (2014)
13. Samuelsson, J., Karlsteen, M., Finnsgård, C.: Differential GNSS for outdoor sports - testing of applicability for alpine sports. In: Proceedings from icSports 2016, 4th International Conference on Sport Sciences Research and Technology Support, Porto, Portugal, 7–9 November 2016, pp. 188–196 (2016). ISBN/ISSN 978-989-758-205-9

Unsubstantial Health and Sports Monitoring Reliability of Commercial Fitness Tracker Bracelets Induced by Their All-in-One Sensing Unit Approach - Experimental Evaluation of Measurement Accuracy in Dynamic and in Steady Physical Effort Scenarios

Hans Weghorn[✉]

BW Cooperative State University, Kronenstrasse 53A, 70174 Stuttgart, Germany
weghorn@dhbw-stuttgart.de

Abstract. The use of electronic tools in medicine and sports is well established fairly long time, because monitoring of physiological body measures like heart rate, effort levels and moving speed parameters supports medical examination as also systematic training control in sports. Fast improvement and miniaturization of computer electronics led to a broad distribution of such technologies not only in professional environments, but also in personal applications like, e.g., tracing fitness activities and endurance workouts in non-elite sports. Since several decades tiny sports watches are available, which are communicating with body sensors and produce with that records of various inputs. The sensing and recording capabilities of such sport tool sets are theoretically also feasible for certain medical applications like, e.g., rehabilitation, because the same physiological measures are of relevance there. Few years ago, yet another device class in the housing style of forearm bracelets came up and was broadly advertised as contribution for supporting a healthier life style. Such units integrate all sensing and control in one single device case, which should make them convenient even for an all-day use. The practical experiments and their analysis, which are reported here, unveil that these bracelet devices cannot sense and record physiological data at an acceptable quality and reliability level, which would be required for using such new unit concepts in professional sports and health tracking or even in rehabilitation and health emergency scenarios.

Keywords: Health monitoring · Sports monitoring · Endurance training · Personal ubiquitous devices

1 Introduction

Considering general health in modern societies, there arise special risk potentials. On the one hand side, our steadily aging citizenships consequence an increased portion of elderly people with naturally higher individual health risks. Especially during the recent decades, it has been investigated and validated in various studies, that physical

© Springer Nature Switzerland AG 2019
J. Cabri et al. (Eds.): icSPORTS 2016/2017, CCIS 975, pp. 55–74, 2019.
https://doi.org/10.1007/978-3-030-14526-2_4

exercises, which are performed on a regular, weekly base, can help people in different problematic fields. For example, stroke risks can be reduced for middle-aged men [1] and women [2]. Same effect is achieved also at higher living ages already by weekly, but extensive walking [3]. Furthermore, it has been investigated and shown, that other health issues can be diminished by following physical workout plans [4].

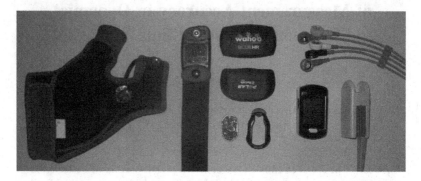

Fig. 1. Examples of sensors for monitoring in health and sports: On the right, an ECG cable set and a pulsoxiometer clip for a clinical patient monitor and one standalone finger pulsoxiometer are visible; in the middle, three heart rate sensors, one with chest contact strap, and the PCB of 3D footpod sensor with shoe clip are shown; on the left, an early glove product for overcoming the chest strap sensing is displayed that is based on optical measurement at the forefinger.

Another aim in recent research and health are concepts for competing growing overweight even from childhood on, which also manifests an increasing issue in modern societies. The impact on healthcare costs has also been repeatedly validated in research [5]. Recent approaches aim, e.g., on how to motivate already children to a daily life with more physical activity. In such concepts, mobile computing with sensing and observation of physiological movements is used quite typically [6].

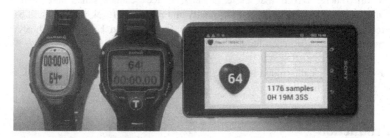

Fig. 2. Sample control units for sports and health supervision: two chest straps with different HR sensors (one ANT+ and one Bluetooth LE), which were attached simultaneously to the same person, feed two sports computers and a smartphone APP with information in parallel. The middle unit marked with T is used in the further investigations here as reference device.

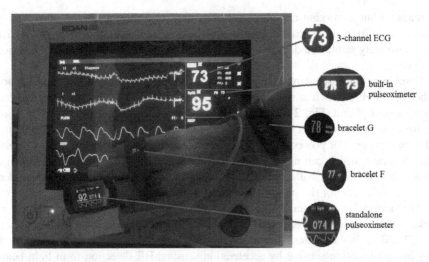

Fig. 3. Using two medical and two bracelet devices for measuring current heart rate: a hospital patient monitor tracks HR by a three-channel ECG and by its wired pulseoximeter at the index finger; bracelet G is worn correctly, while bracelet F is placed incorrectly, and one further standalone pulsoxiometer on the middle finger complements this tracking unit collection.

Such health application scenarios do have close relation to sensing physiological traces of the human body like in controlling sports trainings and competitions. Especially in endurance sports, tracing heart rate (HR) represents a convenient measure [7] for monitoring and control of oxygen balance [8] at an appropriate technical effort. The approach of optimizing HR control in endurance sports and the foundation base behind was discussed already in a project for developing optimized mobile tools for this purpose [9]. Complementing this, the tracking of movement with different types of body motion sensors was evaluated in another study [10].

In medical applications, electrical and optical signal capture of heart beat activities are well elaborated. In particular, HR measures can be derived from a multi-channel ECG or indirectly through optical pulsoxiometer devices (Fig. 1 right part). According to the mandatory quality standards of medical units, the monitoring results can be considered as highly reliable. Sports devices simplified the ECG measuring method to a two-electrode sensor solution with their commercialized chest straps (Fig. 1 middle part). Alternatively, a decade ago, an optical measurement through a glove finger came to market (Fig. 1 left part), which was working similar to the pulsoxiometer concept, but was based on optical reflection from blood-supplied tissue below skin. This system was intended and advertised for overcoming the necessity of HR chest straps, but it didn't persist successfully on the market.

Concerning movement tracing, meanwhile almost any high-end device is using GPS. This, of course, is not working reliably indoor and therefore as complement or as alternative, tread sensors, which were placed as footpod on sports shoes, have been developed and commercialized also since many years (PCB and shoe clip in Fig. 1). There is a clear one-to-one relation between foot stepping and the acceleration sensing in such footpods, hence walking and running parameters like stride rate and total count of treads within a workout can be derived by such sensor units. On the other side, a total moving distance can be only estimated on base of an average foot step with, which is not absolutely stable and depends on the current, particular way and style of walking or running.

Combining these standard technologies in a mobile monitoring device set in sports or health activities, such a system has to consist of typically two or three devices, namely a control unit (Fig. 2) that is linked to the required body sensors (Fig. 1). If an ergometer, a bicycle or other sports machines are used, additional sensors for wheel and pedal turning, and for power output may be present. In sum, a rather complex sensor network forms, which can not really be handled comfortably; it even requires maintenance (e.g. caring for batteries in each single unit) and some technological understanding, especially for the proper placement of all the intelligent sensors.

As comfortable alternative, few years ago wristband devices were brought to market, which should perform the functionality like the before described tool sets (Figs. 3 and 4). In the housing shape of a bracelet, which is worn on the forearm, such units integrate motion sensing by acceleration sensors, HR detection from light beam reflection of skin surface below the device, and also the entire control unit with user interfacing. This means that the units can be easily worn all day - even during sleep - and that is exactly, what they are advertised for by their vendors. From the viewpoint of computer science, the UIs of these devices are rather interesting, because they apply totally new haptic input modes and also some new output technologies, like e.g. organic LED. This enables good case study opportunities of how to interact with the human user more efficiently from very tiny devices.

Compared to the established systems used in medicine and professional and non-elite sports before, these new devices obtain their physiological measurement traces in a more indirect way. Therefore, an experimental study was started for investigating the precision and reliability of this new bracelet fitness tracker class [11]. Here, this study is discussed and re-validated by using in addition a professional patient monitor (Fig. 3) and a set of additional indicative experiments.

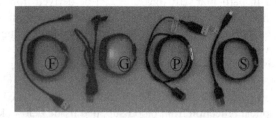

Fig. 4. Four wristband fitness trackers were selected from different vendors, all from a similar price segment. These bracelets are referred in the experiments here with the letters F, G, P and S; all units came with USB cables used for charging and partially also for host communication

2 Experimental Devices

2.1 Hardware Selection

At the time, when the bracelet fitness tracker units appeared on the market, they came up almost simultaneously in a bigger number of variants and from different competing vendors. Some brands were completely new on the market, while other brands were already well established before in the field of commercial sports trackers. For the experimental investigation here, a set of four different devices from separate vendors was selected. The units were taken out of an intermediate price segment, which ranges in the order for sports watch systems with similar capabilities and reputed quality. According to their indication in Fig. 4, these devices are named F, G, P and S throughout this article.

As reference in validating the accuracy and reliability of the bracelets, an expensive, high-ended triathlon sports watch system with HR and tread rate sensor was used, which is called T in the context here (Figs. 1 and 2). Furthermore, a study about reliability of tread sensing devices had been conducted earlier already [10] and it was therefore available as assistive knowledge base. In addition, professional medical devices were selected (Fig. 3) for cross-validation: at first a standalone pulseoximeter was used, which was supplemented in the last phase of this investigation with a medical patient monitor. The latter can measure HR by a multi-channel ECG and is additionally equipped with a wired pulseoximeter. Due to their dimension and handling, these medical devices could only be used indoor.

2.2 Setting up Devices for Operation

While the medical devices and the triathlon computer T can be used completely on their own, bracelets F, G and P can be used only partially standalone. Bracelet S cannot be used at all without RF-coupling it to a smartphone. All bracelets require setup through UIs running on a personal computer (PC) or a smartphone. The construction of the entire bracelet software system bases on a kind of complex device driver software, which is running on the PC and which interacts through a RF link with the bracelet unit. For some units, this communication can be operated alternatively also via an USB cable connection. This software part can be configured by the bracelet user through its own UI, but this method doesn't allow access or inspection of what is happening or has been collected on the fitness wristband.

Accessing any tracking data has rather to be performed through the Web browser on the PC by accessing a tool collection on the Web site of the device vendor. The "device driver" passes all communication from and to the device to mechanisms located on this Web site. This all consequences, that the system can be used only in a very restricted way, if no PC with working Internet connection is available. It further implies that all data is never stored locally and under control and access of the device owner and user, but it is archived on an external server - a method that follows the cloud philosophy approach.

Despite the vendors' claim, that the bracelet user is the owner of all collected data, full access is not possible. Scans can be only displayed through complicate and winding Web UI schemes, which were continuously modified over the entire period of this investigation. Also the software on the wristbands was updated again and again for all the systems. This all suggests that the whole concept and its hardware and software components were released to market at an early and presumably unprofessional engineering stage. The biggest restriction arises from the fact, that the UIs do not give true access to all data scanning points, but they release only summaries of workouts or they show colorful plots, which are breaking the simplest reasonable standards of how to display such function graphs in scientific or technical style.

In particular, one vendor claims that all data can be downloaded to a local PC by the user, but only rough summaries of physical activity traces are made available and no details are accessible like this is easily possible with systems like T. The effort for setting up the entire bracelet software system appears inappropriately high, the rate of required software maintenance over many weeks and months of use can be considered as even worse. The handling of the installation and preparation of unit S appeared more reasonable, which is certainly achieved by fully programmed software with UI, which is running on the local smartphone and which has not to be operated through the limited UI capabilities of Web browsing.

2.3 Features and Feasibility of Operation

After software and device setup, the handling of the bracelets was explored with first, simple tests. While data plots in activity laps collected with F and G could be retrieved through their Web site, this was not possible with device P. Despite all the three other devices, P has no built-in HR sensing, and hence, HR monitoring was not performed with P in this study.

In one of the first, extended experiments, a parallel monitoring with F and G was tested, while device T was used as reference (Fig. 5). During this, F was placed on the left and G on the right forearm of the experimenter. A longer run was broken down into a set of laps for obtaining data sets for a possible statistical evaluation of the tracking measures. For achieving this, the bracelets had to be controlled manually and simultaneously through their mechanical push buttons; this was only possible during intermediate running stops seen as drops in the velocity curve of the test (Fig. 5).

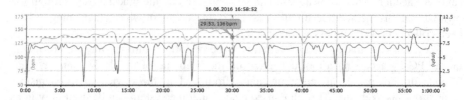

Fig. 5. Reference scan from T for a running experiment shows function plots of HR and moving velocity [11: Fig. 4]; this test was intended for statistically evaluating the measurement quality of bracelet devices F and G that were used in parallel. During the slow down phases, the devices were handled manually for starting and ending the individual laps.

Surprisingly, it turned out during these first examinations, that the UI system of unit F does not release information about the individually recorded laps easily. Further tests with F unveiled, that data plots of individual activity laps only can be inspected on their own, if there is a long time break around a lap of not using F at all. In else cases, the system of F merged all daily activities into one big data scan, making it impossible to derive any statistical evaluation of tracking accuracy. With unit P it was found, that it is impossible to access any activity counts on its Web UI at all. Fortunately, limited lap data sourcing became possible, because all bracelet devices allow displaying their currently collected activity counts directly through their wristband UIs on the devices themselves without using a PC (with the exception of S, which doesn't have any number display). Of course, this working style complicates all experimenting sessions, because continuous breaks for taking handwritten notes are required.

In accordance to these findings, the plan for the original experimental proceeding was therefore revised to the following scheme:

- Only G could be efficiently used to record traces of HR and movement activities with several laps in one compact experimental run.
- F was planned only for single laps in each experiment, at maximum two runs per day seemed possible.
- It was decided to perform most elementary experiments without Web UI for devices F, G, and P by taking handwritten protocols; S was excluded from certain tests, because it lacks an own UI on the wristband.
- Since P does not implement internal HR scanning (RF coupling of a standard chest strap is possible), it was excluded from such tests completely.
- F and G were planed for single, selected activity test laps while recording movement and HR monitoring traces in parallel to T; these should be downloaded later for evaluation from their Web UIs.

3   Measures and Recording Tests

3.1   Scope of Investigation

At the time, when the bracelet fitness tracker units appeared on the market, they came up almost simultaneously in a bigger number of variants and from different competing vendors. For the investigation here, four typical device units from different manufactures were selected to obtain a broader view of the market. The units were selected from a price segment, which ranges within the order for sports watch computer systems from reputed companies providing similar sensor capabilities. In particular, the latter should cover:

- Motion tracking
- Heart rate monitoring

This requirement definition represents the base for efficiently tracing systematic health exercises and activities as also forms a base for efficient sports training and competition control. Therefore, reliability and precision of monitoring of the related physiological measures delivered by the bracelet devices was main scope of a systematic study in this research here.

Concerning motion tracing, meanwhile GPS technology has established itself as standard method. It is available in high-ended sports computers since longer while and allows also to convert modern smartphones, which are equipped with GPS electronics, into a health and sport activity monitor. GPS comes with intrinsic inaccuracy, which is hidden or overcome by signal conditioning algorithms, indoor its functionality is rather limited and on sports machines, like treadmills and ergometers, GPS localization naturally cannot be used at all.

Counting foot steps with acceleration sensors came up as economic solution for motion tracing earlier than GPS, since this could be realized with simple specific devices like pedometers or also with less elaborated mobile phones. Often the thumb rule, that 10,000 steps per day stands for a healthy living style, is cited in various discussion media, but such clear relation lacks of scientific validation [12]. Nevertheless, the method and the devices behind step counting in health and sports applications have been validated in different studies over the years [10, 12]. The fundamental concept and its accuracy limitations are relevant here, because the bracelet units also retrieve their motion tracking in terms of step counting - at least, the devices are exposing measures of this parameter to their users.

For monitoring HR, multi-channel ECG represents the technically established instrument in medicine. Its operation detects activities of the different motor units in the heart muscles with electrical signals on human skin surface. Sports computers use to follow this approach with their HR chest straps, while they try to minimize the number of electrodes in ECG sensing. The alternative technology with optical sensing of HR is also available in medicine as side measure in pulsoximeter sensing, and it is the key concept, which is applied in the bracelet fitness trackers.

In the experiments here, particular aspects should be investigated systematically in respect to monitoring physiological activity parameters:

- Reliability of tracking
- Average accuracy and variance of measures

Before performing such use tests of the devices, their physical dimensions were measured. Table 1 shows a comparison of the four experimental bracelet units with the established electronic tools. The wristband trackers have only a clear size and weight advantage, if they are set into relation to the high-ended other units. Compared to more simple systems from sports electronics, the bracelet weight and size is not considerably smaller.

Table 1. Measures of physical dimensions for different tracker devices.

	Sports watch		Smartphone		Bracelet			
	T	Simple	Sports	Full + slim	F	G	P	S
Weight [gram]	73	43	113	132	28	31	28	27
Size [cu. cm]	35.0	15.8	79.2	77.3	9.24	11.34	7.80	7.33

3.2 Motion Tracking by Means of Step Counting

The systematic investigation of the reliability and precision of the bracelet trackers in motion tracking was performed in two stages. As measuring base, walking and jogging is applied, because this stands for activity in health [1–3, 12] and sports [10].

Table 2. Registration values as displayed by the bracelet devices during the manual counting experiments with 100 full walking steps.

Bracelet	F	G	P	S
Synchronous arm swing	167	203	200	180
Damped arm swing	203	203	150	152

At first stage, tests were performed how bracelet trackers register foot steps at all. Variation during walking and running is possible by moving the arms in different manner, either with a natural swing that is synchronized to the foot moves or in a damped way, where the arms are kept intentionally close to the body with the aim of avoiding too much of arm oscillation. Table 2 lists the results for the four tested devices. It can be derived, that for an average user it remains unclear, how to move in a way, that all devices F, P and S all count properly. Only G appears insensitive against the arm moving style in walking.

This first experiment proves, that most of the bracelet units are unable to register each individual foot step reliably like this is known from devices, which are worn inside a shoe - like the sports acceleration sensors - or close to the body like mobile phones inside a pocket or pedometers [10, 12]. An average user will move the arms unconsciously and without specific control, which means there will be a linear mixture of precisely and imprecisely counted steps. Assuming equal distribution between these two cases, a measurement error of approximately 10% can be expected, especially if the foot steps are converted to a moving distance as discussed in experimental stage two in this section. Another extreme observation about device S has to be added here also: while the behavior exposed in Table 2 was stable for device F, G and P, unit S produced a variation in its count value of 80% during the synchronous arm swing, when these step registration experiments were repeated several times.

Table 3. Verification, whether typical gym workouts incur false step counting (sets of 20 repetitions each were repeatedly conducted).

Bracelet	F	G	P	S
Squats	Counted	Counted	No	Counted
Dumbbell front raise	Counted	No	Counted	Counted
Dumbbell lateral raise	Counted	No	No	Counted
Arm circling	Counted	Counted	Counted	Counted

The second part in the first test stage about counting reliability was to test, whether and how step counts are registered in the devices, if the user is not walking. Also when a person is not walking, there will be arm moves during all the occupation in daily life, hence the possibility arises that acceleration sensors on the forearm misinterpret such movements as foot stepping action. Similarly, gym exercises are based on controlled arm moves without walking. Table 3 lists test results, whether the bracelet units are registering such activities as walking steps. Units F and S produce 100% errors in this, while G and P come here with a chance of 50% faulty counting. The result from this test series is the proof, that all bracelet units are registering step counts from arm movements despite no foot steps are preformed. This stands for another, important effect of unreliable step counting.

In the second stage of the movement tracing investigation, a set of lap measures for registered moving distances should be recorded during jogging. From this, a statistical evaluation of tracking precision should be derived. Devices P and S had to be excluded from these tests, because covered distances can not be retrieved neither from these devices themselves nor from their host UIs. Also the Web UI of device F doesn't allow to record and display a set of laps individually, but test on movement tracking could be performed by manually handling this bracelet through its one button input and its built-in LED screen. In this way, it was possible to manually read the actual step counting and total distance on F's tiny number display.

Table 4. Hand written protocol for unit F in tracking ten times a moving distance of 0.5 miles; w_n list the result for walking laps @3.5 mph approx., while j_n list jogging laps @6.5 mph.

Lap no.	w_1	w_2	w_3	w_4	w_5	J_1	j_2	j_3	j_4	j_5
Steps [counts]	928	422	873	924	898	779	774	773	777	776
Distance [miles]	0.43	0.19	0.41	0.43	0.43	0.47	0.46	0.46	0.47	0.46

For the experiments with F and G a straight path was chosen, which is located parallel to the river Danube. A suitable segment of 0.5 miles was selected along the official river landmarks, which are placed there every 200 m. This path length was validated additionally by a GPS trace and with a bicycle computer, which measures elapsed distances from wheel turns.

Device F was used in a series of five walking laps and five jogging laps there (Table 4), while after completion of each lap the intermediate step counting values and the elapsed distances as displayed on the wristband were written on paper. Table 4 shows, that during jogging unit F has got a high repetition quality and a systematically too low distance measure, while walking imprecision and unreliability of unit F appears much increased.

Furthermore, it turned out as side observation in the test series of Table 4, that device F registered finishing of floor levels while moving the arm up and down for reading the values from the display. This suggests that the floor level counting is also performed in a nonsensical way, and its result is worthless. Another side observation was, that unit F produced a buzzing applause when reaching approximately 6.4 miles in a longer test run. With this, unit F aimed to congratulate for just collecting 10,000 foot steps, which was clearly wrong and much too high, because the food stride length in the applied way of jogging was known from the experiments in [10] and didn't map to the total distance at this point. Despite the displayed distances show only a smaller error, the step counting of F works considerably incorrect and imprecise as seen in stage one already.

Step counts of a workout can be converted by a certain factor, which is determined as average foot step size, into the total covered distance. In sports computers, which use to function according to this concept, it is possible to calibrate or to program the step width. This was not possible with the here used software versions of the bracelets. Accordingly, it was not possible to achieve correct distance tracking, even if the step counting would work precisely.

In contradiction to the situation with the other wristbands, the Web UI of device G lists all individual laps out of one bigger activity as these are launched and terminated through the manual bracelet input. Figure 6 shows a set of five lap runs on the 0.5-mile path, the image is a fraction of the entire Web UI screen for G. Figure 7 lists the results for these laps from reference device T, which were recorded in parallel to G. From this data collection it can be derived, that G registers covered distances systematically too high. In consequence, the moving speed also is reported wrong proportionally.

Activity Type	Start ▾	Distance	Time	Avg Speed(Avg Pace)	Max Speed(Best Pace)	Avg HR	Max HR
Running	Thu, 16 Jun 2016 5:49 P...	0.59	4:23	7:29	5:22	146	151
Running	Thu, 16 Jun 2016 5:38 P...	0.58	4:27	7:38	5:29	142	148
Running	Thu, 16 Jun 2016 5:27 P...	0.59	4:30	7:37	4:57	141	146
Running	Thu, 16 Jun 2016 5:16 P...	0.57	4:23	7:40	3:31	139	145
Running	Thu, 16 Jun 2016 5:06 P...	0.58	4:25	7:37	5:23	139	144

Fig. 6. This table is the part of the entire Web screen display for device G, which lists five consecutive test run laps; each lap had a three times validated length of 0.5 miles.

For unknown reasons, the Web UI of G did not show the counting totals for foot steps in this experiment, so it cannot be validated, whether the distance error refers to a wrong step length parameter, which also cannot be calibrated in this device. There is a time gap of approx. one minute between the recordings of device G in Fig. 6 and T in Fig. 7, but T works with GPS and must be therefore absolutely precise.

In summary, the movement distance tracking for jogging activities can be considered as comparably precise to the method based on the footpod sensors despite the movement is detected by the bracelet on the forearm, which does not have a 1:1 relation to foot stepping. This concept suffers anyway from an intrinsic problem, because in general step width is a varying value and not a fixed parameter. On the other hand, in an all day use or for some devices in walking, false step counts can be accumulated and will produce big errors in the reports about daily activity sums. The bracelet measures use to feed the illusion, that the device owner is much more active than what is reality fact.

17:07:10	0.50 mi	4:23.30	8:50 /mi	6.8 mph	7.5 mph	140 bpm	144 bpm	87 U/Min.
17:17:04	0.50 mi	4:21.62	8:46 /mi	6.8 mph	7.7 mph	141 bpm	145 bpm	85 U/Min.
- 17:28:46	0.50 mi	4:28.91	9:01 /mi	6.7 mph	7.5 mph	142 bpm	145 bpm	85 U/Min.
- 17:39:00	0.50 mi	4:25.64	8:54 /mi	6.7 mph	7.6 mph	143 bpm	147 bpm	86 U/Min.
- 17:49:52	0.50 mi	4:21.54	8:46 /mi	6.8 mph	7.3 mph	147 bpm	150 bpm	88 U/Min.

Fig. 7. The PC software for triathlon sports computer T provides complete information for any workout instantly: these text lines, which are fragments from the entire UI screen display of T, show the reference recordings, which correspond to the five test laps with G in Fig. 6. This data validates that G registers covered distances systematically too high.

3.3 Heart Rate Monitoring

The wristband trackers F, G and S read the heart rate from a light beam, which is reflected from skin surface on the forearm under the devices. This realizes a fundamentally different detection method than known from the electrical sensing in medical ECG and HR chest straps in sports computers like T. For exploring the efficiency of this HR reading concept, use modes with almost constant heart rate and with varying heart rate were applied. This is achieved by steady physical effort levels like in endurance workouts, and by dynamic effort demands, e.g. during sets of gym workouts with intermediate breaks. The latter testing was performed already before in [11] with consecutive sets of arm stemming.

This kind of examination was re-validated with another experiment in this extension of the whole study, where T again was used as reference device and wristbands F and G were recording simultaneously HR traces: after a resting phase of 5 min, which included preparation of the gym activity, four sets of combined squats and overhead handle pushes were conducted. The last set was performed with breath holding for provoking higher variation in HR, recovery phases were applied between the repetition squat/handle raise sets.

Reference device T is equipped with a barometric altitude sensor; it was attached to the weight handle during the entire time of the test. Therefore, the recorded activity curves in Fig. 8 for unit T indicate the active phases in the altitude measure, while the HR trace shows the low level of 58 bpm during the initial resting phase and the count of 113 bpm at a time point of 8 min 45 s for the maximum HR in the whole workout. The recordings for F and G show, that these devices cannot follow dynamics in HR. Only during the resting phase, these wristband units produce reasonable HR measures. This new test confirms the findings reported in [11: Fig. 3] about the weaknesses in HR traces by F and G.

In the steady effort scenarios of endurance training, the wristband G shows in Fig. 6 comparable, but not precisely exact measures for HR average and HR maximum. Again reference was taken by T in this set of 5 test laps (Fig. 7). Since device F does not allow retrieval of individual running laps, F should be used in one of the test examinations only in just one single out of a set of several experimental laps, which was performed with devices F, G, and T in parallel. As reported in [11: Fig. 5], the finding arose, that F invents HR data randomly, when it is detached from the body. This kind of fraudulent behavior was also detected by another wristband model sold by the

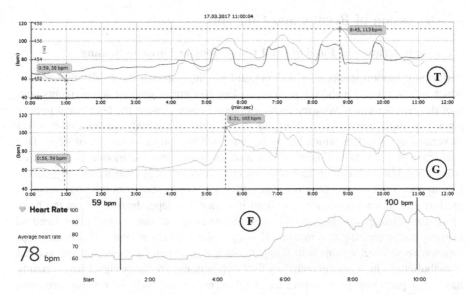

Fig. 8. After a resting phase, the experimenter stood up and performed four sets of 20 squats with parallel overhead handle stemming. Reference unit T was attached to the handle, its recordings show accordingly the physical activity phases in the barometric altitude measure and the HR scan with its resting value and maximum count. Wristband units G and F can yield only reasonable HR measures during the initial resting phase, while both trackers are totally incapable of following dynamics in the physiological input signal of HR properly.

vendor of F in the frame of validation experiments for an on-going PhD thesis about health emergency scenarios. Since it is impossible to determine, when F truly measures HR data and when it invents such measures blindly, no further statistical evaluation about its accuracy was performed.

In summary on HR sensing, it can be stated that both wristbands appear not feasible for dynamic scenarios at all. If HR would stay stable for a longer while at the same level, these devices may measure this physiological parameter with acceptable accuracy. Unfortunately, this situation is rarely found in true-world use cases. Even in long endurance workouts, sports people use to apply pickup training parts, where HR changes. Many physiological exercises in health and sports base on the variation of effort level and by that on the variation of HR, because else there won't be good training effects. Also the advertised idea for the wristbands of detecting restless phases during sleeping will not work well, because health problems like sleep apnea provoke also sudden increase of HR, which cannot be detected by the wristbands. In general, any human activity will be an unknown mixture of steady and dynamic HR phases, therefore the risk is always present, that the bracelet units will generate unreliable and imprecise output, if they are applied for the purpose of HR tracing or monitoring, regardless whether this refers to health or sports use cases.

4 Discussion of Results and Concepts

4.1 Consideration of Fundamental Limitations in Forearm Sensing

Performing motion tracking in walking and jogging through an acceleration sensor, which is worn inside a shoe, represents a clear concept of relating sensor inputs with foot stepping activities. Wearing an acceleration sensor close at the body torso implies already first indirection, because up and down moves of the body are detected in terms of vertical acceleration, which has to be translated into an estimate of foot steps. This concept was used by pedometers and also in sports apps of mobile phones quite reasonably, but with certain and nominal error bars [10, 12]. The wristband trackers add another level of indirection, because they are worn away from the body torso on the forearm. Since human arms are used in a totally independent way from the body torso, the sensing unit is exposed to a considerably increased number of freedom degrees in acceleration and motion. Hence, in the forearm position the sensor reads superimposed acceleration from independent arm and hand actions and the vertical contributions, which are generated by foot step actions. The latter signal part certainly has got a particular profile, because the landing of the body in running produces typically short and strong breaking forces of up to three times earth gravity. Unfortunately, this is not strict and varyingly lower, if a person is just walking. Hence, successful signal de-convolution requires a high signal-to-noise ratio and a very good knowledge base about acceleration curve profiles. Tables 2 and 3 show that this can not be fulfilled systematically, and a wide range of errors in foot step detection is preprogrammed by this concept of foot motion detection at forearm position.

From medical devices the weak signal-to-noise ratio in optical sensing of heart beats from skin is known from the typical behavior of pulsoximeters. At measurement start, such devices typically require a longer series of cycles, until they can synchronize themselves to the pumping blood flow and produce results. Despite such sensors work with a light beam shining through the finger and their position is fixed with a clamp, any tiny finger movement of the measurement apparatus cause disturbances in the input signal curve and distorts the measurement (sample visible as background curves in Fig. 2). The sports glove with the modified optical concept of sensing the light from reflection instead of transmission, which was introduced approximately a decade ago, hasn't been a success, because it was unreliable. Since the wristband trackers work also on base of sensing of reflected light from skin surface, and since their position is not fixed in the optimal forearm position, it could be expected, that the concept cause problems. In accordance, the experiments have shown the effect of measurement delays, if there is a slope in HR. How often the input signal is lost during normal use is not known, because the devices interpolate results in such cases, which has been proven by intentionally interrupting the reflection beam. It can be expected, that problems with detection occur continuously during arm movement and by that during any physical activities in general.

4.2   Evident Self-protection of Bracelet Vendors

Devices like S indicated partially from the beginning in their user manuals, that they are not feasible for medical purposes. Meanwhile this instruction is presented more clearly during installation phase of the software systems. Other devices like F and G continuously present in their Web UIs links with a note about sensor quality, while the information behind explains that the user cannot rely on the collected data. The intense of such advices has increased during this study, which is now running over ca 1.5 years and this information policy can be presumed as reaction to the fact, that worldwide many people and institutions sued some of the bracelet vendors because of the objection between product advertisements and delivered quality.

Like in [13], users quickly detected the obvious sensing quality lack of wristband trackers and put a mass of critical reports in feedback sites of Internet selling platforms. The reaction pattern of the device manufactures appears simple: instead of improving their devices, they simply claim that the devices are not reliable, of course this restriction is neither visible on the selling packages of the units nor in advertisement media presentations like TV promotion spots. This represents a modern style of tricking customers by fine print information with the primary intent of selling a mass of units also at a low state of product quality and reliability.

For adding a remarkable benefit of the wristband devices although the main purpose of sports and health monitoring is not fulfilled, some vendors provide features of using the units for remote control and remote display of the user's smartphone, e.g. in messaging and performing phone call. With respect to the primary and advertised sense of the device as fitness monitor, adding such functionalities seem to represent a kind of displacement activity in developing fully functional consumer electronics.

4.3   Possible Positive Impact of Wristband Fitness Trackers

Despite all critical findings about the functionality and reliability of the bracelet trackers, there arise also some positive effects due to their plain existence. Since big marketing campaigns were launched by the vendors for the new tracker concept in various broadcasting media, it can be considered as assured that more people were attracted for the topic of health and an improvement of daily living style. Especially advertisement campaigns, which are launched repeatedly before celebration events - presumably with the intent of offering bracelet fitness trackers as possible present for relatives and friends -, keep the awareness of a healthy and sports-oriented daily living style alive. This was also detected and taken into advantage by some companies, who have strong interest in sustaining a healthy way of living of their employees, as samples like [14] demonstrate. Using the bracelets as indicator will help motivate company people to participate such community activities regardless how precise the devices are in reality.

Another positive aspect is that bracelet units with their limited size and input possibilities enable an exploration field for new, appropriate UI concepts for such very tiny units. According to the experience with the tested units here, a superset of new UI modes can be applied and tested for its feasibility:

- Device detects arm move, e.g. towards face ⇔ automatic switching-on of display helps saving electrical energy and yields implicit handling convenience.
- Sensitivity and reaction to finger touches and swiping in different directions and styles (linear or circular) provide a huge set of additional input modes.
- Single (mechanical) button control in terms of short, long and quick multiple press also provide different modes of user input communication.
- Exploring readability of new output electronics like organic LEDs, especially when exposed to daylight.

These UI modes are totally new in comparison to traditional workstations handling with keyboard and pointing device, which also differs considerably from the use of smartphones and electronic tablets. Such concepts and ideas are also highly required due to the very limited surface size of such units. The high amount of units on the market and their broad use will provoke technological darwinism, through which the most convenient and efficient UI handling modes with very tiny devices will be selected.

4.4 Summary on Current Usability and Improvement Concepts

Utilization of the fitness tracker bracelet leads to a high consumption of time, which is not directly related to their main purpose. This effort has to be spent at several software levels; again and again upgrades either of the bracelet firmware or other components are required during daily use. The systems are following the cloud concepts by enabling an access to collected workout data only through Web sites, which is time-consuming and inefficient. Without Internet access, the bracelet devices can be used only in a very limited way; privacy and security concerns arise from the fact that user data is stored in a place, which is not under control of the customer and where rules can be changed any time by the device vendor.

Concerning quality of the core functionality of the wristbands, experimental results have shown in this study that the HR forearm sensing concept is extremely unreliable; it is presumed, that this arises from fundamental limitations in the applied optical beam detection from skin reflection. Even more fraudulent software mechanisms in the wristband trackers, which report measures despite there is no way of obtaining them, exclude such units from reasonable applications and demote the bracelets below quality of toys. Figure 9 exposes another sample of such tricky constructions, which can be read certainly also as irresponsible and disrespectful to customers, who are willing to pay money for such systems and can therefore expect certain performance.

Activity tracing in terms of counting foot steps, covered distances and other parameters do indeed work to some extend at a quality level, which is known from other comparable systems like pedometers and sports computers. Devices like G demonstrate, that step counting in sports activities like walking and jogging can work sufficiently on base of forearm sensing, only calibration would be required to improve the concept. Other bracelet units behave not as efficient, and all wristbands suffer from unreliable measurements, if the type of moving activity is not know by the device or differs from jogging. This suggests that if the current use mode of the wristband is defined in an on-going measurement and accounted in the software, typical precision in motion sensing could be achieved by appropriate algorithms.

Therefore, the existing technology provides enough bases for a valuable wristband tracker concept. For instance, the handling of the device can be optimized by using the OLED display concept, which is well readable also at daylight and by using haptic device input control by arm raises. In combination, various input modes from touch screen swipes would enrich communication between the tiny device and the user considerably. One mechanical button appears sufficient for making input actions clear, also modes of long, short and multiple presses allow variation in control through this single button. Such ideas can be also applied into the other direction of communication, the wristband can inform the user by short, long and chopped mechanical vibrations about various situations, e.g. that a lap or workout is completed or that the user should adopt effort level in an ongoing workout. In other words, combining all positive UI concepts from the existing bracelets of the different vendors into just one wristband and leave away the adverse UI elements, like tiny and weakly shining displays, would lead to a construction that can be handled very conveniently.

Since there will always remain limitations in the direct UI handling of the wristband device, a host like a PC or - as a modern style solution - a smartphone with a handling software app, which directly communicates with the wristband, would be the next requirement stage of improvement. Through this, workouts could be prepared for instance by setting up a lap sequence with certain goals (e.g. time, number of steps, map to HR range, or similar) and the collected data can be inspected directly, even a life screen of the physiological measures could be mirrored on the bigger UI. This all is missing in the current host handling mechanisms for the wristband devices.

With such direct controls, it would also be possible to inform the wristband about the actual activity and on base of this, improved and more reliable step and movement tracking would be enabled as explained before. In this sense, the wristband could truly replace other trackers with their additional motion sensors. If HR should be measured really by the wristband, it has been shown that this is not working continuously in a reliable way. A possible solution would be, if the bracelet informs the user at certain times, e.g. every hour in a health monitoring application, that a measurement should be performed and that the user should assist with keeping the forearm still and the device in optimal position.

The alternative is to interlink the wristband tracker with other HR sensors of high quality and reliability, in particular HR chest straps from sports. Exactly this is done by device P, and for G it is offered as alternative HR tracking to the built-in sensor. As even more radical concept the wristband could be reduced to a remote display device, which communicates with another main tracker system, for instance a smartphone, which is located close to the body and which uses own - and if applicable other - sensors for reliably and accurately detecting physiological measures. Such a concept has been reported already in [9], but with a wristband unit that looks more like a clock. Exactly in this sense, the wristband unit could be constructed even more lightweight and tiny, and by that lift out its main purpose of improving user handling in terms of comfort and convenience in health and sports monitoring.

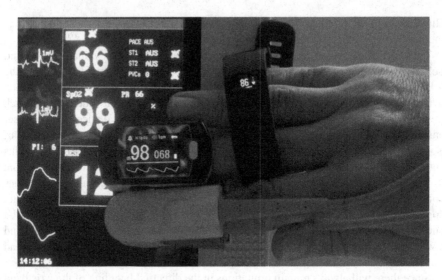

Fig. 9. In this experiment, bracelet unit F was worn intentionally incorrect: despite detached from body skin, it displays blindly a heart rate of 86 BPM, while the three simultaneous medical measures mutually validate a true count that is considerably lower.

5   Conclusions

Aging societies and a widely distributed unhealthy life style in our modern societies pose new questions and challenges for appropriate compensation concepts. Already since many decades, computer electronics is widely established as supporting technology in medical environments as also in professional and personal health and in sports applications. In particular, mobile patient monitors are commonly used in medical investigation and the same applies for handheld sports computers, which are interlinked with a sensor network for tracing the physiological body state. These are commonly used even in non-elite sports, especially like running and cycling.

The required wiring or the attachment and maintenance of various body sensors like chest straps with heart rate sensors, are often experienced as uncomfortable. Extended use of such devices like, e.g. wearing a long-term ECG measuring unit, is sensed as really uncomfortable and therefore is acceptable only for a limit time span despite these tools are designed as being mobile. A new device concept, which came up few years ago, seemed to overcome these concerns with a much improved handling convenience. Integrating all sensing and electronics in one single casing, which is worn as bracelet on the forearm, was introduced and advertised as comfortable solution for an all-day monitoring opportunity of physiological body measures. This surveillance ranges from resting phases while sleeping to intense effort levels like during, e.g., demanding endurance activities.

Meanwhile, it has been suggested already from a broader mass of user experience reports, which can be sourced from the feedback on Internet shop platforms, that these bracelet units do not fulfill typical demands for data quality in physiological sensing of body activities. In accordance to such non-scientific notes, the experimental study here, which was conducted with cross validation by medical device units and high-ended professional sports computer systems, has shown that bracelet data is not only randomly inaccurate, it has been proven that these devices even use to invent sensor data, when signal sourcing verifiably is lost. The latter applies in particular over extended time spans. Of course, such fraudulent mechanisms exclude affected wristband trackers from any use, where reliability and accuracy is mandatory. The all-in-one sensing concepts appears being a clear fail, which is not too surprising in respect to the well-known foundation bases in physics and medicine.

In the end, feasible devices in medicine, health and sports are available and can be used together efficiently with their multi-sensor body networks. Recent evolvements of the bracelet units also employ established and reliable technologies like GPS localization and RF-coupled sensors, so the trend is that newer bracelets contain the original technical solution of sport watch computers, which is just put into a different housing style. This necessary dissociation from the all-in-one unit brings back all the inconvenience, which should be overcome with the wristband construction. Certainly, the appearance of the bracelet units on the market and the big advertisement campaigns helped to make people more aware about healthy behavior and inspired people to be more active on various levels in daily life. Also for computer scientists the tiny devices manifest an experimental ground for the improvement of UI concepts with very tiny devices, which stands also for some positive impact of such units.

References

1. Abbott, R.D., Rodriguez, B.L., Burchfiel, C.M., Curb, J.D.: Physical activity in older middle-aged men and reduced risk of stroke: the Honolulu Heart Program. Am. J. Epidemiol. **139**(9), 881–893 (1994)
2. Oguma, Y., Shinoda-Tagawa, T.: Physical activity decreases cardiovascular disease risk in women. Am. J. Prev. Med. **26**(5), 407–418 (2004)
3. Jefferis, B.J., Whincup, P.H., Papacosta, O., Wannamethee, S.G.: Protective effect of time spent walking on risk of stroke in older men. Stroke **45**, 194–199 (2014)
4. Law, M.R., Wald, N.J., Meade, T.W.: Strategies for prevention of osteoporosis and hip fracture. BMJ **303**, 453–459 (1991)
5. Colagiuri, S., et al.: The cost of overweight and obesity in Australia. Med. J. Austr. **192**(5), 260–264 (2010)
6. Valentín, G., Howard, A.M.: Dealing with childhood obesity: passive versus active activity monitoring approaches for engaging individuals in exercise. In: Biosignals and Biorobotics Conference (BRC), 2013 ISSNIP, Rio de Janeiro, Brazil, pp. 166–170. IEEE Press, New York (2013)
7. Arts, F.J., Kuipers, H.: The relation between power output, oxygen uptake and heart rate in male athletes. Int. J. Sports Med. **15**(5), 228–231 (1994)
8. Kindermann, W., Simon, G., Keul, J.: The significance of the aerobic-anaerobic transition for the determination of work load intensities during endurance training. Eur. J. Appl. Physiol. **42**, 25–34 (1979)

9. Weghorn, H.: Application and UI design for ergonomic heart rate monitoring in endurance sports: realizing an improved tool for health and sports activities on base of android smartphone programming and ANT+. In: Cabri, J., Pezarat Correia, P., Barreiros, J. (eds.) icSPORTS 2013. CCIS, vol. 464, pp. 25–41. Springer, Cham (2015). https://doi.org/10.1007/978-3-319-17548-5_3

10. Weghorn, H.: Accuracy evaluation of commercial motion sensing devices in respect to health activity monitoring concepts. In: IADIS International conference e-health 2014, Lisbon, Portugal, pp. 271–278. IADIS Press (2014)

11. Weghorn, H.: Experimental investigation of the usefulness of bracelet trackers in sports and health monitoring - critical evaluation of a new handheld activity monitoring device class. In: 4th International Congress on Sports Science and Technology Support icSPORTS 2016, Porto, Portugal, pp. 124–133. Scitepress (2016)

12. Tudor-Locke, C., Basset, D.R.: How many steps/day are enough? Preliminary pedometer indices for public health. Sports Med. **34**(1), 1–8 (2004)

13. Van Arsdale, A.: Not the ideal Heart Rate tracking tool, March 2015. https://www.amazon.com/gp/review/R15S3GDU59CQ02?ref_=glimp_1rv_cl. Accessed 03 Sept 2017

14. Barker, L.: Fitness trackers: helpful or just hype? In: Dallas News, March 2014. http://www.dallasnews.com/life/healthy-living/2014/03/24/fitness-trackers-helpful-or-just-hype. Accessed 03 Sept 2017

Space Sports – Sailing and Equestrian Sports in Space

Maria Sundin[1,2], Lars Larsson[1,3], Christian Finnsgård[1,4(✉)], and Petra Andersson[5]

[1] Centre for Sports Technology, Chalmers University of Technology,
Gothenburg, Sweden
christian.finnsgard@chalmers.se
[2] Department of Physics, University of Gothenburg, Gothenburg, Sweden
[3] Department of Mechanics and Maritime Sciences,
Chalmers University of Technology, Gothenburg, Sweden
[4] SSPA Sweden AB, Research, Gothenburg, Sweden
[5] Department of Philosophy, Linguistics and Theory of Science,
University of Gothenburg, Gothenburg, Sweden

Abstract. Sports in space? Is it at all possible to practice sports in our solar system but not on Planet Earth? Mars is our closest neighboring planet, and Titan is the largest moon of Saturn, and apart from the Earth it is the only body in our solar system where a liquid exists on the surface. Within the last ten years a system of lakes and rivers has been discovered. The climate and seasonal cycles of Titan are still not very well known, but the composition and pressure are fairly well established. Perhaps in the future boats will sail the lakes of Titan for research purposes or even sport.

The purpose of this paper is to give an overview of the concept of space sports, looking at sailing on Titan and equestrian sports on Mars. For sailing, the conditions of Titan necessitate calculations of important parameters of sailing such as floatability, stability, hull resistance and sail forces. This paper shows that if a sailing yacht on Titan will have twice as large displacement as on Earth and it will be 2.6 times less stable for the same beam. Since friction will be smaller, it will be faster than on Earth at low speed, but significantly slower at high speeds due to the wave generation. The same sail area is required to get the same sail forces if the average wind is 3 m/s, while a 9 times larger sail area is required if the wind speed is only 1 m/s.

Equestrian sports on Mars could be a possibility, even if challenges exist in form of a cold climate and thin atmosphere with noxious gases. Due to the lower gravity sports such as show jumping, dressage and races would yield new records and new patterns of locomotion.

Keywords: Space · Titan · Mars · Sports · Sailing · Equestrian sports · Hydrodynamics · Ethics

© Springer Nature Switzerland AG 2019
J. Cabri et al. (Eds.): icSPORTS 2016/2017, CCIS 975, pp. 75–85, 2019.
https://doi.org/10.1007/978-3-030-14526-2_5

1   Introduction

Today the International Space Station has been manned since the year 2000. Serious plans of sending humans to Mars in the near future exist, indeed it has recently been decided to be a priority goal for NASA. The European Space Agency is discussing having a manned base on the Moon by 2030. Perhaps humanity one day will colonize a large part of our solar system. The idea of sports then being practiced in space is probably not too strange. Space Sports would be performed under very different conditions than Earth Sports, and completely new possibilities would arise.

Sports research indicate new records being harder and harder to obtain in some sports. Possibly, the limits of human capability for certain sports as well as horse capability for the equestrian sports will soon be reached. But, one could argue, only on this planet! On other planets it might be possible to jump higher and patterns of locomotion and the motion of objects will differ. Earth Sports could be adapted and new sports could be created. Could interplanetary championships exist? Could an athlete from Earth compete against an athlete from Mars? How, and on which planet in that case?

There are a large number of sports that could be investigated using physics and technology. How high could a horse jump on Mars, how fast can it run, how extraordinary hind leg movements can it perform? Can you sail on the lakes of Titan, the largest moon of Saturn? How large would a goal in soccer have to be on the moon? Can you fly using muscular power on Pluto? What is the pattern of locomotion when running in a different gravity? Is The Jovian moon Europa the perfect place for skating? How do you play ball in zero gravity? Can you ski on Olympus Mons, the highest mountain in the solar system?

The number of possible questions about space sports are almost endless. This paper introduces one concept study of space sports by looking at sailing on Titan and equestrian sports on Mars.

2   A Brief Overview of Our Solar System

Our sun is a medium sized yellow star, one of the approximately 200 billion stars in the Milky Way galaxy. Around the sun there are eight planets and minor bodies such as dwarf planets, moons, asteroids and comets.

The planets are usually divided into two separate categories; terrestrial planets and gas giants. The terrestrial planets are Mercury, Venus, Earth and Mars in order from the sun and outwards. The gas giants are Jupiter, Saturn, Uranus and Neptune. Terrestrial planets are substantially smaller than the gas giants with the diameter of Jupiter being 22 times larger than the diameter of the Earth. Rocks and metals are the main constituents of the terrestrial planets, while the gas giants have large layers of hydrogen, helium, ices and hydrocarbons in different states surrounding rocky cores.

The distance between the Earth and the sun is some 150 million km, and this distance is usually referred to as 1 Astronomical Unit (1AU). Mars is located at 1.5 AU, so the four terrestrial planets are fairly close together when it comes to astronomical distances. Jupiter is at 5.2 AU from the sun and the outmost planet Neptune is at 30 AU.

Most of the bodies of the solar system orbit the sun in the same plane, the only exception being the large spherical cloud of comets surrounding the sun at the outskirts of our solar system.

3 Liquids on Planetary and Lunar Surfaces

Oceanus Procellarum – Sea of Storms, Mare Crisium – Sea of Crises, Mare Tranquillitatis – Sea of Tranquillity and Mare Imbrium – Sea of Rains.

The names of the dark areas on the moon are most likely exciting for any sailor. Indeed, their names reflect a time when they were mistaken for being oceans and seas instead of the dry lava plains we now know them to be. No liquid water can exist on the surface of the moon primarily due to the absence of an atmosphere.

Large amounts of liquids on the surface of a planet or a moon is in fact extremely rare in our solar system. Titan, the largest moon of Saturn, is probably the only place excepting our own Earth. The seas, lakes and rivers of Titan are however not filled with water but the hydrocarbons methane and ethane in liquid state.

Since Titan then is the only other body in our solar system with a liquid on the surface, it is also the only other place where we could practice sailing. Will we ever do that, and why in that case?

Most likely the first expeditions to Titan would be for scientific purposes much like the way we are exploring Mars today. The exploration of Mars is partly being done using robotic rovers, and on Titan robotic boats could be an option. A great advantage of sailing is it being a form of transport without the need of extra energy sources. In space exploration, energy is always one of the limiting and costly factors.

The research on autonomous vehicles on the Earth is evolving rapidly, and autonomous boats on Titan would be an enormous advantage since the communication time between the earth and Titan is an approximate hour. NASA is currently discussing the possibility of sending a submarine to Titan.

Of course, the possibility exists of Titan being colonized in the future. Manned sailing boats could then become reality and apart from transport perhaps even sailing could become a recreational pleasure as well as a sport.

Why then are the Earth and Titan the only bodies in our solar system with liquids on their surfaces? The uniqueness of Titan is the conditions being right for the existence of a relatively thick atmosphere. A certain atmospheric pressure is necessary for the existence of liquids instead of having a substance in solid or gaseous state. The surface pressure on Titan is larger than on the Earth, and the atmosphere of Titan consisting mainly of nitrogen.

Our neighbor planet Mars has such a thin atmosphere that liquid water can hardly exist on the surface anymore. Large amounts of water are present on Mars, but almost all the water is in solid state (ice) with the transition to water vapour being very quick when heated. The lack of atmosphere on Mars is due to a weak gravity and no shielding magnetic field. The solar wind is a stream of electrons and protons from the sun, and it exerts a pressure on the Martian atmosphere. On Earth our atmosphere is partly shielded by our magnetic field. The weak Martian gravity has not been able to hold on to the originally much thicker atmosphere when battered by the solar wind.

Jupiter and Saturn are our two largest planets and they are called gas giants. Both have more than 60 moons each. Several of these moons are exciting worlds in different sizes and with varied surfaces. A few of the moons are actually larger than the planet Mercury. A planet moves around the sun, and a moon moves around a planet but planets and moons can be of equal sizes. Titan is the second largest moon in our solar system, but it is smaller than Mars in both radius and mass. Why then has Titan not lost its atmosphere when Mars has? The reason is it being much colder out by Saturn at 9.5 AU than at Mars at 1.5 AU. The average temperature on Titan is around −180°. This will lead to the velocities of the molecules in the atmosphere not being as high. It is easier for the gravity to hold on to a cooler gas than a hot one, since fewer of the molecules reach the escape velocity. Titan is also shielded from the solar wind by the magnetic field of Saturn.

Already in the 1980's the speculations of lakes on Titan began triggered by data from the Voyager space crafts. When the Cassini space craft arrived after a ten-year long journey in 2004 hopes were high of a rapid detection of the lakes. But it took three more years until the lakes were finally proved to exist in 2007. Today we know that the largest lake of Titan Kraken Mare has a surface of 400 000 square kilometers and a depth of 160 m. Its surface is probably just a little bit smaller than the surface area of Sweden and possibly larger than the Caspian Sea. Titan has several other lakes and rivers of different sizes and depths and shows an intriguing landscape. Measurements so far indicate flat lakes and low velocities of the winds, but modelling of Titans climate shows possibilities of strong winds and even hurricanes. This has received support by other studies of the landscape.

Saturn orbits the sun with a period of approximately 29 years. The seasons are therefore some 7 years each. When Cassini reached Saturn in 2004 the northern hemisphere of Titan was in deep winter. Now, fifteen years later the northern hemisphere is approaching the summer solstice. This means that we have not as yet had the opportunity to study the climate of Titan during a whole "Titan-year". Therefore, it is quite uncertain how valid the weather observations are when it comes to average conditions.

4   The Possibility of Sailing on Titan

So, what are the possibilities of sailing on Titan, and how different would it be from sailing on Earth? Would it be at all possible, and what would the boats look like? To assess the possibilities we need to consider aspects like floatability, stability, hull resistance and sail forces.

These properties are in turn dependent on physical constants like the density and viscosity of the atmosphere and the liquid, and on the gravity. Wind speed is of course also an important parameter. In Table 1 the physical constants are listed, based on data from Cassini. For comparison, the corresponding values on the Earth are also presented.

Table 1. Physical constants [1].

Constant	Titan	Earth
Atm. density, ρ_a [kg/m^3]	5	12
Atm. viscosity, v_a [m^2/s]	1.3×10^{-6}	15×10^{-6}
Liquid density, ρ_l [kg/m^3]	530–660	1030
Liquid viscosity, v_l [m^2/s]	0.3×10^{-6}–3×10^{-6}	10^{-6}
Acc. of gravity, g [m/s^2]	1.4	9.8

Let us start with the floatation, i.e. how deeply the boat will float in the liquid. The gravity force F_G (downwards) is obtained as (from [11]):

$$F_G = mg \qquad (1)$$

where m is the total mass of the boat and g is the acceleration of gravity. The buoyancy force, F_B (upwards) is equal to (from [11]):

$$F_B = \rho_l D g \qquad (2)$$

Where ρ_l is the liquid density and D is the submerged volume (*displacement*) of the hull. This is according to Archimedes' principle. At equilibrium (from [11]):

$$F_G = F_B \qquad (3)$$

which yields (from [11]):

$$D = m/\rho_l \qquad (4)$$

Since g appears both in F_G and F_B it disappears from the final equation, which says that for a given mass the displacement is inversely proportional to the fluid density. According to Table 1 the density on Titan is about half of that on Earth. Therefore the displacement will be twice as large on Titan as on Earth for a given mass. Stability is of fundamental importance for a sailing yacht. As appears from Fig. 1, it is achieved through the sideward movement to leeward of the centre of the underwater volume from B to B' when the yacht heels [2].

Since F_B acts at the centre of buoyancy, it will create a righting moment with F_G. A vertical line along F_B will cut the heeled center plane of the yacht at the metacenter, M. The distance between this point and the centre of gravity G is called metacentric height and is denoted $\overline{GM}$. It follows that the righting arm, RM, can be computed as $\overline{GM} \sin \phi$, where ϕ is the heel angle, and that the righting moment, RM, is (from [11]):

$$RM = F_G \overline{GM} \sin \phi \qquad (5)$$

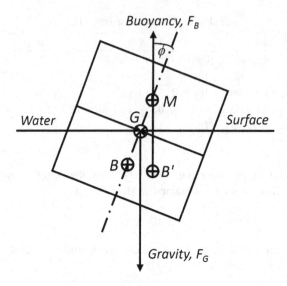

Fig. 1. Stability principle [11].

To compute the righting moment we need the metacentric height $\overline{GM}$. This can be computed using the distance from B to M, $\overline{BM}$, which is obtained from a fundamental formula in stability theory [2]

$$\overline{BM} = I/D \tag{6}$$

where I is the moment of inertia around a longitudinal axis of the area inside the waterline of the hull.

For a sailing yacht, B and G are close together and $\overline{BM}$ and $\overline{GM}$ are approximately equal. With this approximation, and using (1) for the gravity, the righting moment is (from [11]):

$$RM = mg \sin \phi I/D \tag{7}$$

For a given mass and heel angle the righting moment is thus proportional to g and I/D. As seen in Table 1, the gravity on Titan is seven times smaller than that on Earth, so for the same stability I/D has to be 7 times larger. Now, for a given length, the inertia I is proportional to beam cubed, while the displacement D is proportional to beam to the first power. It follows that I/D is proportional to beam to the second power. For I/D to be 7 times larger than on Earth beam has to be increased $\sqrt{7}$ times, i.e. about 2.6 times.

A hull with the same length as on Earth, but twice as beamy would satisfy the displacement criterion above but it would be less stable. To remedy this, the hull could be longer and it could carry more ballast. The main parameter of interest may be the payload the yacht can carry. For a given displacement this depends on the weight of the yacht itself. The heavier the yacht, the smaller the payload. The weight increases with beam, but much more so with length. So from this point of view it is better to make the hull wider. This will however increase resistance, as we will see. Another very interesting possibility is to use a catamaran. Then stability is no problem and the resistance low.

Having considered the most important properties, floatability and stability, we now turn to the speed potential of the yacht. This is determined by the driving forces on the sails and the resistance of the submerged part of the yacht. Let us start with the latter.

There are two main components of resistance for a body moving along the surface of a liquid: friction and wave resistance. The former occurs because of the internal friction in the fluid, its viscosity, while the latter is caused by the generation of waves transmitted from the body.

Similarity laws for scaling resistance [3] show that friction, R_F, may be computed as (from [11]):

$$R_F = C_F 0.5 \rho U^2 S \tag{8}$$

where C_F is a friction coefficient, ρ the fluid density U the fluid velocity and S the wetted surface of the body. C_F is determined by the Reynolds number, R_n (from [11]):

$$R_n = UL/v \tag{9}$$

where L is a characteristic length of the body and v the kinematic viscosity of the fluid.

Table 1 gives a range of possible viscosities for the liquid on Titan. The range is however centered around the value on Earth (10^{-6} m^2/s). Since the dependence of C_F on R_n is essentially logarithmic [3] it is enough for the present discussion to note that the order of magnitude is the same for the liquid viscosity on Titan and Earth. We can thus assume the same C_F. For a given speed, friction is then proportional to ρS. As we have seen the density on Titan is half of that on Earth, but the wetted surface is larger if the hull is made twice as wide. However, not so much that it compensates for the lower density. Friction may thus be assumed somewhat smaller on Titan.

As shown in [3] the wave resistance is governed by the Froude number, F_n.

$$F_n = U/\sqrt{gL} \tag{10}$$

Neglecting some higher order effects, a constant Froude number will imply the same wave pattern (scaled with length) and the same wave resistance coefficient, C_W, regardless of the speed, length and gravity. The wave resistance, R_W is obtained from the coefficient in the same way as the friction in Eq. (8) (from [11]):

$$R_W = C_W 0.5 \rho U^2 S \tag{11}$$

Unlike C_F, C_W will not be the same as on Earth. This is for two reasons. A wider hull will give a larger C_W, and, more importantly, a given speed will give a higher Froude number on Titan, thereby increasing C_W. The first effect can be roughly estimated as proportional to beam, i.e. for double beam a twofold increase for a given Froude number. But the second effect is difficult to estimate. The relation between C_W

and F_n. is very nonlinear, and also dependent on the hull shape. For most standard yachts there is a maximum Froude number around 0.45, where the wave resistance gets so large that the driving force from the sails is insufficient for increasing the speed. This limit will now occur at $\sqrt{7}$ times smaller speed than on Earth, due to the 7 times smaller gravity (see Eq. 10). In fact the whole wave resistance/speed curve will be compressed in the speed direction by a factor $\sqrt{7}$.

At low speeds friction dominates over wave resistance and, as seen above, the speed may then be somewhat larger on Titan, but at higher speeds the total resistance depends mainly on the wave resistance, and then the speed will be considerably smaller due to the Froude number effect.

Finally, let us look at the sail forces. The sail is a wing which generates a force with components in the direction of motion, F_x and at right angles to that, F_y. Both can be obtained in a similar way as R_F and R_W (both from [11]):

$$F_x = C_x 0.5 \rho_a V^2 S_s \tag{12}$$

$$F_y = C_y 0.5 \rho_a V^2 S_s \tag{13}$$

where C_x and C_y are coefficients ρ_a the density of the atmosphere, V the wind speed and S_s the sail area. Like for the liquid, the coefficients depend on the Reynolds number (from [11]):

$$R_{na} = VC/v_a \tag{14}$$

where C is the mean chord of the sail and v_a is the kinematic viscosity of the atmosphere.

The wind speed on Titan is not well known. There are indications of occasional hurricanes, but the normal wind speed should be quite low. According to Habib the average speed is estimated to about 3 m/s. Other sources quote lower speeds, around 1 m/s [1, 4]. On Earth the average wind speed is 6.6 m/s [5].

Let us first assume a wind speed of 3 m/s. As seen in Table 1, the atmospheric viscosity on Titan is about 1/10 of the viscosity on Earth, so the Reynolds number according to Eq. (14) is about five times larger for a given sail. This yields a slightly lower friction coefficient on the sails, but this will have a very small effect on the forces, which are almost exclusively caused by pressure differences between the two sides of the sail. We can thus assume that both C_x and C_y are the same on Titan and Earth for a given sail. Equations (12) and (13) then show that the forces are proportional to ρV^2. Table 1 shows that the atmospheric density on Titan is about four times that on Earth, but on the other hand, the wind speed is only about half in our assumption. So ρV^2 turns out to be the same! The sail forces will thus be unchanged.

The other scenario with an average wind speed of 1 m/s will yield 9 times smaller forces! To get the same sail forces on Titan as on Earth the sail area has to increase 9 times!

A factor speaking in favour of the lower wind speed is that no waves have been observed on the lakes of Titan. This may however be a matter of measurement accuracy [1]. If the wind speed is only 1 m/s very small waves will be generated and they will not influence performance. However, if the speed is 3 m/s the waves could be significantly larger than the average on Earth. This is due to the fact that the forcing of the waves, pressure variation in the atmosphere, is the same, as we have seen, but the gravity and density of the fluid lower. Such large waves will slow down a sailing yacht considerably, at least sailing upwind.

5 The Possibility of Equestrian Sports on Mars

The whole idea of colonizing other planets of course gives raise to several ethical questions. Questions about risks, precaution and consequences, among others, both regarding the humans that are sent to other planets and the other planets as such, have been discussed [6, 7, 8, 9 and 10].

Here, we leave the ethical considerations on humans colonizing other planets. One can ask why we should bring animals, horses or other, to other planets. One can also ask whether it can be justified to bring horses to other planets. To get the first question in its proper perspective, we can try to turn it around. Why would we not bring animals to other planets.

From ethical and existential aspects, are there several good reasons to bring animals when colonizing other planets. Not only from the resource perspective. Even if we all are vegetarians, we still need fertilizer to farm.

As human beings, Homo sapiens, we have been living close to domestic animals for thousands of years and we have obviously been surrounded by animals for all our existence on Earth. It is even hard to imagine humans living without animals around. No birdsong, no butterflies, no dogs that wags the tails. The question why bring animals to other planets is almost like asking why we should bring each other. New research shows that human history along with domestic animals is longer than previously thought. People also have independently domesticated animals in different parts of the world about the same time.

Human-animal relationships are also healthy for humans, and an important part of human welfare. From an existential point of view, we all see ourselves and talk about ourselves as human beings. Why – and how - should we even talk about humans, if there were no other species (that are relevant to us)? We talk about humans and horses in order to point out particular species, certain forms of life. It seems meaningless to talk about humans - Homo sapiens - if human is the only species available, as it is meaningless to talk about horses - Equus caballus - if that is the only species available. To sum up, the reasons for bringing animals – horses – when colonizing other planets are – beside the need of manure for farming – that animals promote human health in several aspects and also most plausible promote human self-knowledge, just by being others lifeforms and as such they are both contrasts and mirrors to our existence.

What it would mean to live without being able to create relationships with other living beings than other people, almost defies the imagination. The animals are so intertwined in our cultural history that we can hardly imagine culture without them. What is a statue of a king on his horse without a horse? Common sayings like "dog is man's best friend" will lost its meaning if there are no dogs. Bringing horses when we colonize Mars, making it possible for us to keep in touch with a lot of our earthly history and ourselves, one could argue.

Ethics, though, is not only about human and humanity. There are also different theories in animal ethics, making animals into ethical subjects, not only as manure delivering tools for farming. Can it ever be ethically justified to bring horses to other planets? How will horses handle the environment when moved so far from the planet where they evolved?

There are large differences between the Earth and Mars. The average temperature on Mars is around −50 °C. Variations in temperature exist since, just like the Earth, Mars has seasons. During favorable conditions the temperature might rise to +20 °C in some regions. This climate is probably more troublesome for humans than horses, because horses are comfortable at lower temperatures than humans are. In addition, horses deal more effectively with cold than humans, just by eating more. Hence, the cold on Mars is not necessarily a reason not to bring horses there. Already on Earth, it is usual to protect horses from cold, rain and wind with the help of rugs. These rugs are already available in different qualities for different weather and temperatures.

Astronauts quickly learned that the moon requires a different movement pattern than they were used to from walking on Earth, because of the lower gravity. On Mars the gravity is more than twice as high as the Moon, but it still probably requires that horses adapt their movements. That opens for new and so far, unseen opportunities in equestrian sports. The Martian gravity can be calculated from the mass and size of Mars resulting in a value of 37% of the Earths. When jumping, a horse can therefore probably rise its centre of mass 2.7 (1/0.37) times higher than on the Earth. Grand Prix obstacles could be 4.5 m high! Perhaps the horses perceive the higher obstacle like a wall. These new conditions may also lead to new knowledge about training horses and about trust between man and horse. How do we get the horse so confident that it jumps over an obstacle that is higher than the horse itself? The trust between rider and horse will be tried, and that will also give new opportunities to learn new things about the relationships between species, e.g. human and horse. Dangerous and even mortal accidents is unfortunately part of the equestrian sports. One positive effect of the lower Martian gravity would be a lower risk of being injured when falling off a horse.

Horsepersons are extremely interested in their patterns of locomotion, their gaits. The horse's movements determine how much we can hope for the individual horse in terms of results in competitive equestrian sports. The quality of the horse's movements is attributed great importance in the horse's utility as sport horse and the horse's economic value. We do not know how the horses will react to the lower gravity, and how they will adapt their movements but this would change sports such as dressage. Most likely, changes in bone mass and muscles would occur in a horse in a similar way to what astronauts subject to lower gravity for long times experience. The future gaits of a Martian horse are therefore hard to predict.

Finally, the atmosphere of Mars is very thin and consists almost only of carbon dioxide. One future possibility is buildings and larger areas with domes containing breathable air. Another solution could be riders and horses carrying breath masks and tanks filled with air when moving on the Martian surface.

6 Conclusions

Titan is the largest moon of Saturn, and apart from the Earth it is the only body in our solar system where a liquid exists on the surface. Within the last ten years a system of lakes and rivers has been discovered. The climate and seasonal cycles of Titan are still not very well known, but the composition and pressure are fairly well established. Perhaps in the future boats will sail the lakes of Titan for research purposes or even sport. This paper addressed some of the issues that will have to be considered before sailing on Titan, or even designing a boat for sailing on Titan's lakes.

A sailing yacht on Titan will have twice as large displacement as on Earth, it will be 2.6 times less stable for the same beam. Since friction will be smaller, it will be faster than on Earth at low speed, but significantly slower at high speeds due to the wave generation. The same sail area is required to get the same sail forces if the average wind is 3 m/s, while a 9 times larger sail area is required for if the wind speed is only 1 m/s. To avoid the stability problem a catamaran seems to be a good choice!

If Mars will be colonized by humans in the future, we might bring animals. Equestrian sports could be a possibility even if challenges exist in form of a cold climate and thin atmosphere with noxious gases. Due to the lower gravity sports such as show jumping, dressage and races would yield new records and new patterns of locomotion.

Acknowledgements. The authors wish to acknowledge the support from Chalmers Area of Advance Materials Science, and the Department of Physics of University of Gothenburg. And Västra Götalandsregionen via Regionutvecklingsnämnden for its financial support.

References

1. Hayes, A.G., et al.: Wind driven capillary-gravity waves on Titan's lakes: hard to detect or non-existent? Icarus **225**, 403–412 (2013)
2. Larsson, L., Eliasson, R.E., Orych, M.: Principles of Yacht Design. Adlard Coles Ltd., London (2014)
3. Larsson, L., Raven, H.C.: Ship Resistance and Flow, PNA Series. Society of Naval Architects and Marine Engineers, Jersey City (2010)
4. Bird, M.K., et al.: The vertical profile of winds on Titan. Nature **438**, 800–802 (2005)
5. Habib, M.: Let's put a sailboat on Titan (2015). www.universetoday.com/111216/lets-put-a-sailboat-on-titan
6. Sparrow, R.: The ethics of terraforming. Environ. Ethics **21**(3), 227 (1999)
7. Otto, E.: Kim Stanley Robinson's Mars trilogy and the Leopoldian land ethic. Utopian Stud. **14**(2), 118 (2003)
8. Pinson, R.: Ethical considerations for terraforming Mars. Environ. Law Report. **32**, 11333 (2002)
9. Schwartz, J.: On the moral permissibility of terraforming. Ethics Environ. **18**(2), 1–31 (2013)
10. York, P.: The ethics of terraforming. Philosophy Now: A Magazine of Ideas, October/November 2002
11. Sundin, M., Larsson, L., Finnsgård, C.: Space sports – sailing in space. In: Proceedings from icSPORTS 2016 on 4th International Conference on Sport Sciences Research and Technology Support, 7–9 November 2016, Porto, Portugal, pp. 141–146 (2016). ISBN/ISSN: 978-989-758-205-9

Construction and Validation of Protocol for Digital Measurement of Human Body

Igor Gruić[1(✉)], Darko Katović[1], Anita Bušić[2], Tomislav Bronzin[3], Vladimir Medved[1], and Marjeta Mišigoj-Duraković[1]

[1] Faculty of Kinesiology, University of Zagreb, Zagreb, Croatia
`igor.gruic@kif.hr`
[2] Live Good j.d.o.o., Zagreb, Croatia
[3] Citus d.o.o., Zagreb, Croatia

Abstract. Standardized measurement protocol for assessing anthropometric dimensions of human body is precisely predefined by International Biological Programme (IBP), [16]. Objective of this research was to produce, compare, validate and standardize protocol for digital measurement (DM-I) using Kinect sensor in order to economize future large scale research. Results in selected variables revealed that classically and digitally measured parameters, e.g. *height*, in average results do not differ significantly, while e.g. for lengths of the left forearm and the left lower leg do indicate lower values. Different reference points used in two measurement methods, i.e. anthropometric points (IBP) and Kinect points, represent similar, but not identical representation of human body. Measures of internal consistency (reliability) for assessed digitally measured variables demonstrated high reliability, but inappropriateness for clinical trials demanding extremely high precision. Since reliability of instruments in clinical and sport application differ, broad spectrum of useful specific diagnostic tools and instruments may be produced based on results assessed in this research.

Keywords: Anthropometry · Reliability · Kinect · Protocol

1 Introduction

Anthropometry (from Greek ἄνθρωπος *anthropos*, "human", and μέτρον *metron*, "measure") refers to measurement of certain human being [16].

"Within biomechanical and healthcare communities, reliable estimates of body segment parameters (BSPs) are desirable for a number of analyses. For example, calculation of body volume index (BVI) is reliant on accurate measures of segment volume, whilst inverse dynamics models require estimates of segment mass to calculate joint force and power. Accuracy is paramount, as small changes have been shown to greatly influence subsequent calculations" [4]. According to Katović et al. [12], various methods of human body assessment use various instruments. In the fashion industry, a common instrument is the measurement tape, while in biomedical sciences anthropometric instruments include: anthropometer, pelvimeter, calliper, centimetre tape, etc. Digital measurement methods for human body assessment use various electronic systems (e.g. Kinect, Structure Sensor). These methods range from laser scanners to

© Springer Nature Switzerland AG 2019
J. Cabri et al. (Eds.): icSPORTS 2016/2017, CCIS 975, pp. 86–99, 2019.
https://doi.org/10.1007/978-3-030-14526-2_6

mobile applications (e.g. Tailor Measure and Nettelo). Three-dimensional scanners enable innovative and quick digital anthropometric measurements based on gathered information from sensors, e.g. Kinect sensor. Microsoft Kinect is used in the field of anthropometrics [4, 22, 24, 29, 30], gait analysis [2, 18, 20, 21, 27], motor performance [13, 25, 28], posture/balance training [7, 15, 19, 23] and rehabilitation [6, 9, 17, 26].

The goal of this research was to initially determine reliability of instruments in clinical and sport trough validation of a new measuring instrument for digital measurement of anthropometric dimensions of the body (structural and metric), to determine the Kinect anthropometric measurement error based on comparison with classical anthropometry, and the optimal distance between a subject and the Kinect sensor, etc.

2 Methods

Sample of n = 52, male and female, employees of Technology Park Zagreb, voluntarily joined the classical (on a smaller scale measures) and digital (in the full range of measures) measurement of anthropometric dimensions in their own clothes with long sleeves and trouser

2.1 Variables

Among 471 assessed variables (3 + (26 * 6) * 3) three variables from a set of classically measured anthropometric dimensions were extracted - *height, length of left forearm* and *length of left lower leg*. Classical measurement procedures for assessing anthropometric dimensions were carried out according to the pre-defined and standardized IBP (International Biological Program) protocol [16].

Standardized measurement protocol for digital measurement of anthropometric dimensions, using a device, was defined via equipment, procedures and instructions, controlled during measurement of each entity for full control of factors that may affect the accuracy of measurements (Figs. 1, 2 and 3).

Classical Anthropometric and Kinect Measurement Protocols
Standardized measurement protocol is predefined by IBP. Standardized protocol for digital measurement (DM-I) was [12]: *Run time:* The total estimated duration of the test for one subject is 6-8 min. *Number of measurers:* 2. *Technical requirements:* A computer with configuration: 64-bit (x64) dual-core, 3.1 GHz or faster (Intel i3, i5 or i7), USB 3.0 controller dedicated for Kinect v2 sensor (Intel chipset), 4 GB of RAM, the graphics card that supports DirectX 11, Windows 8, 8.1 or Windows 10, and Kinect version 2 for Windows. *Description:* The test was performed in a room with minimum dimensions 3 × 4 m. Kinect and computer device were on the table 75 cm high, with lines showing distance of 200 cm, 230 cm and 260 cm from the Kinect (a tape on the floor that followed an imaginary line perpendicular to Kinect). *The initial position of the examinees:* The subject stands upright in a straddle stand facing the measuring instrument, feet spread at hips-width and rotated outward (V-position). The hands are placed parallel to the trunk and away from it forming a 35–45° angle. Examinees' approximated mean normalized distance between top and middle of human head) view

Table 1. Examples of comparison of measures and terminology of IBP and MS Kinect.

Br.	IBP	Kinect points (from – to)
1	Body Height	Head to Foot
2	Left Upper Leg Length	Hip Left to Knee Left
3	Left Upper Right Length	Hip Right to Knee Right
4	Left Lower Leg Length	Knee Left to Ankle Left
5	Right Lower Leg Length	Knee Right to Ankle Right
6	Left Leg Length to Ankle	Hip Left to Ankle Left
7	Right Leg Length to Ankle	Hip Right to Ankle Right
8	Left Leg Length to Foot	Hip Left to Foot Left
9	Right Leg Length to Foot	Hip Right to Foot Right
10	Hip Width	Hip Left to Hip Right
11	Shoulder Width	Shoulder Right to Shoulder Left
12	Torso Height	Spine Base to Spine Shoulder
13	Neck Height	Neck to Spine Shoulder
14	Face Height	Head to Neck (+10 cm)
15	Left Forearm Length	Wrist Left to Elbow Left
16	Right Forearm Length	Wrist Right to Elbow Right
17	Left Upper Arm Length	Elbow Left to Shoulder Left
18	Right Upper Arm Length	Elbow Right to Shoulder Right
19	Left Hand Length	Hand Tip Left to Wrist Left
20	Right Hand Length	Hand Tip Right to Wrist Right
21	Left Arm Length	Shoulder Left to Hand Tip Left
22	Right Arm Length	Shoulder Right to Hand Tip Right
23	Arm Span	Hand Tip Right to Hand Tip Left

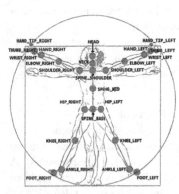 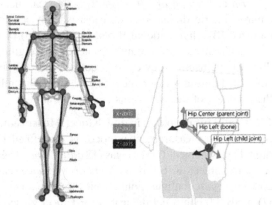

Fig. 1. Measurement points recognized by Kinect v2 sensor (Left ankle, Right ankle, Left elbow, Right elbow, Left foot, Right foot, Left hand, Right hand, Tip of the left hand, Tip of the right hand, Head, Left hip, Right hip, Left knee, Right knee, Neck, Left shoulder, Right shoulder, Base of the spine, Middle of the spine, Spine at the shoulder, Left thumb, Right thumb, Left wrist, Right wrist).

Fig. 2. Measurement points recognized by Kinect v2 sensor represented on human skeleton.

Fig. 3. Basic calculation of distance between calculated measurement points (Microsoft Kinect v2 sensor calculates Head point as a central point of head surface in height of centre of nose with additional 10 cm added, which represents.

was focused straight ahead in the direction of measuring device. The proper starting position and distance of subjects from instrument was checked by measurer before issuing instructions to start with protocol. *Measurement of performance:* After coming into the position to measure, participants were supposed to raise their left arm, which starts the process of positioning the object of measurement by the device. After dropping an arm and coming into the initial default position, measurer activates measurement procedure, and an examinee retains position until next instructions. The task was performed six times on each of three default distances. Between individual attempts, examinee has to leave the position and to come back. *Completion of performance measurement:* The task is completed when the subject performs six registered measurements on each of the three default distances. *Position of measurers:* The first measurer was in a position that allows him to control the position of the examinee in the measurement, visual inspection of the task and the registration results. Another measurer enters codes of each measurement in a prepared table. *Recording the results:* The device automatically registers the default digital (anthropometric) measures (3 × 6 measurements) in centimetres (with a precision of 1 decimal). After each measurement, measurer records identification number of a measurement in the prepared table. *Remark:* The examinee may begin the process of positioning at any time, raising his left hand after he was warned by the measurer that the instrument is ready. If the result wasn't registered for any reason, measurement procedure must be repeated. *Information to the examinee:* [task was demonstrated and described simultaneously] "This protocol measures the dimensions of your body. To start measuring, your task will be, after taking a starting position at a given distance, to raise and lower the left arm. Stand upright, facing the screen of the monitor, with eyes directed forward. The arms are slightly separated from the body, extended at the elbows, fingers outstretched and hands in continuation of the extended forearm." (Measurer demonstrates the position of the body and at the same time describes) "The task will be repeated six times, on each of the pre-set distances. On the measurer's sign, after each recorded measurement, you will leave your position and return back. Is your task clear? Take the starting position and prepare for measurements."

2.2 Statistical Analysis

Data were analysed by Statistica 12.7 for Windows operating system. Mean, standard deviation, range, variability coefficient, skewness and kurtosis were used as descriptive parameters, supported by the Pearson correlation coefficient, Cronbach's alpha and Spearman-Brown (standardized) alpha in validation analysis and the average inter-item correlation.

3 Results

Average results of digitally measured heights compared to classically measured heights do not differ significantly, which were followed by the standard deviation values (Fig. 4), the coefficient of variation and form of distribution parameters (Table 2).

Table 2. Descriptive parameters for variables height, left forearm and left lower leg [12].

	Mean.	Std. dev.	Minimum	Maximum	Range	VarCoef	Skewness	Kurtosis
A_Height	176.41	8.19	159.00	192.30	33.30	4.64	−0.14	−0.30
D1-[1]	177.06	8.12	160.46	197.69	37.23	4.59	0.07	0.05
D2-[1]	176.10	8.48	159.50	197.89	38.39	4.82	0.11	0.05
D3-[1]	176.11	8.31	159.13	196.92	37.80	4.72	0.04	−0.06
A_L_fore arm	26.94	1.77	23.10	30.70	7.60	6.57	0.07	−0.15
D1-[15]	23.92	1.40	21.35	26.47	5.12	5.87	0.01	−0.63
D2-[15]	23.77	1.48	21.00	26.38	5.38	6.21	0.02	−0.84
D3-[15]	23.56	1.55	20.33	28.42	8.08	6.59	0.45	0.98
A_L_lower leg	39.36	2.71	32.60	46.30	13.70	6.89	−0.08	0.07
D1-[4]	35.11	2.59	30.18	41.32	11.13	7.37	0.16	−0.03
D2-[4]	34.93	2.35	30.32	42.00	11.68	6.72	0.24	0.50
D3-[4]	35.74	2.38	30.40	41.30	10.90	6.67	−0.07	−0.15

A_height Standard measured height, D1-[1] Digitally measured height at distance of 200 cm, D2-[1] Digitally measured height at distance of 230 cm, D3-[1] Digitally measured height at distance of 260 cm; A_L_forearm Standard measured length of left forearm, D1-[15] Digitally measured length of left forearm at distance of 200 cm, D2-[15] Digitally measured length of left forearm at distance of 230 cm, D3-[15] Digitally measured length of left forearm at distance of 260 cm; A_L_lower leg Standard measured length of left lower leg, D1-[4] Digitally measured length of left lower leg at distance of 200 cm, D2-[4] Digitally measured length of left lower leg at distance of 230 cm, D3-[4] Digitally measured length of left lower leg at distance of 260 cm.

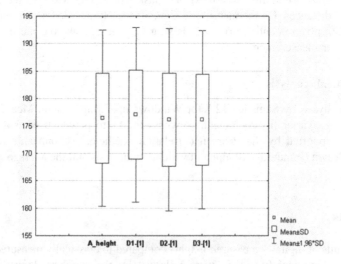

Fig. 4. Descriptive parameters for variable height [12]; **A_height** Standard measured height, **D1-[1]** Digitally measured height at distance of 200 cm, **D2-[1]** Digitally measured height at distance of 230 cm, **D3-[1]** Digitally measured height at distance of 260 cm.

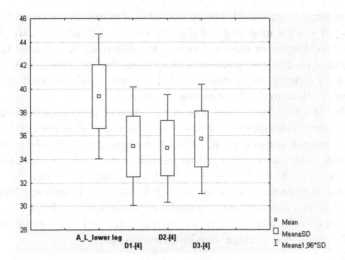

Fig. 5. Descriptive parameters for variable left forearm length [12]; **A_L_lower leg** Standard measured length of left lower leg, **D1-[4]** Digitally measured length of left lower leg at distance of 200 cm, **D2-[4]** Digitally measured length of left lower leg at distance of 230 cm, **D3-[4]** Digitally measured length of left lower leg at distance of 260 cm.

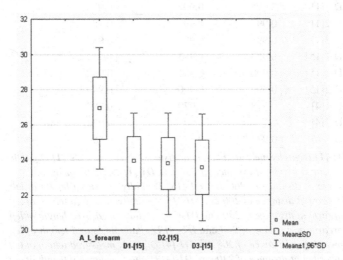

Fig. 6. Descriptive parameters for variable left lower leg [12]; **A_L_forearm** Standard measured length of left forearm, **D1-[15]** Digitally measured length of left forearm at distance of 200 cm, **D2-[15]** Digitally measured length of left forearm at distance of 230 cm, **D3-[15]** Digitally measured length of left forearm at distance of 260 cm.

The descriptive parameters of variables - *left forearm length* and *left lower leg length* (classically and digitally measured), indicate significant differences (lower values) between average results digitally measured in relation to results in the classically measured variables (Table 2). The value of parameters of standard deviation (Figs. 5 and 6) and the total range of digitally measured results are lower than classically measured lengths of the left forearm. The difference is attributed to different reference points used in two measurement methods. For periphery of human body, indirectly, it is contrary to Clarkson et al. [4] where results showed that the 3D scanning system 'systematically overestimate volume'.

Reliability of a new digital measuring instrument was determined by the method of internal consistency (appropriate for this type of composite measuring instrument). Measures of internal consistency for digitally measured variables: *body height, left forearm length* and *left lower leg length* (measured six times at each of three distances - Table 3) demonstrate high reliability. (Cronbach alpha, the standardized alpha 0.995 to 0.997) and the average inter-item correlation (0.973 to 0.985), indicate a high internal consistency between items related to digitally measured heights (Table 3). Reliability coefficients for digitally measured left forearm and lower leg lengths was slightly lower (greater differentiation in average inter-item correlations).

Table 3. Coefficients of reliability for variables height, left forearm and left lower leg [12].

	Cronbach alpha	Standardized. alpha	Average inter-item correlation
D-1[1]	0.995	0.995	0.973
D-2[1]	0.997	0.997	0.985
D-3[1]	0.997	0.997	0.985
D-1[15]	0.983	0.983	0.914
D-2[15]	0.990	0.991	0.952
D-2[15]	0.990	0.990	0.949
D-1[4]	0.978	0.979	0.887
D-2[4]	0.987	0.988	0.932
D-3[4]	0.97	0.97	0.886

D1-[1] Digitally measured height at distance of 200 cm, ***D2-[1]*** *Digitally measured height at distance of 230* cm, ***D1-[1]*** *Digitally measured height at distance of 260* cm, ***D1-[15]*** *Digitally measured length of left forearm at distance of 200* cm, ***D1-[15]*** *Digitally measured length of left forearm at distance of 230* cm, ***D1-[15]*** *Digitally measured length of left forearm at distance of 260* cm, ***D1-[4]*** *Digitally measured length of left lower leg at distance of 200* cm, ***D1-[4]*** *Digitally measured length of left lower leg at distance of 230* cm, ***D1-[4]*** *Digitally measured length of left lower leg at distance of 260* cm.

Simulation of the possible impact of reduced number of items indicated a decline of reliability (e.g. in digitally measured height at a distance of 200 cm, and after removing the last 3 items, Cronbach alpha reduced its value to 0.987). Same simulation for digitally measured left forearm length revealed a value reduction of Cronbach alpha from 0.9777 to 0.952, which could consequently result in an increase of the standard error of measurement.

Reliability tested in Clarkson et al. [4] revealed that the relative technical error of measurement has shown to be on average 0.88% (±0.1). Relative accuracy was quantified by calculating intraclass correlation coefficients, which was found equal to 0.997 for the 3 repeated scans across all assessed participants.

Analysis of differences between the descriptive parameters (Table 4) of classically and digitally measured variables (body height, left forearm length and left lower leg length), reveal the size of systematic and non-systematic errors and its effect on measurement results. Increased variability (standard deviation, total range, coefficient of variation) indicate a presence of large quantities of non-systematic errors probably caused by technical/environmental factors. Differences in heights and left forearm lengths increase by distance, while differences in lower leg lengths relatively decrease in variability by an increase in distance.

Table 4. Differences in descriptive parameters for variables height, left forearm and left lower leg [12].

	Mean.	Std. dev.	Minimum	Maximum	Range	Var Coef.	Skewness	Kurtosis
d1_height	0.66	2.78	−5.39	6.60	12.00	420.46	0.06	−0.34
d2_height	0.05	2.89	−7.38	5.59	12.96	6448.31	−0.11	−0.01
d3_height	−0.35	3.06	−6.53	5.33	11.86	−884.48	0.02	−0.69
d1_L_forearm	−3.04	1.14	−5.57	−0.87	4.70	−37.37	−0.40	−0.15
d2_L_forearm	−3.14	1.21	−7.12	−0.92	6.20	−38.55	−0.89	1.45
d3_L_forearm	−3.38	1.48	−7.22	−0.48	6.73	−43.77	−0.70	0.54
d1_L_lower leg	−4.25	2.31	−9.93	2.72	12.65	−54.38	−0.16	1.37
d2_L_lower leg	−4.35	2.18	−10.22	3.40	13.62	−50.08	0.18	3.54
d3_L_lower leg	−3.66	2.13	−9.20	2.92	12.12	−58.16	0.06	1.40

d1_height – variable of difference between digitally and standard height measure at distance of 200 cm, d2_height – variable of difference between digitally and standard height measure at distance of 230 cm, d3_height – variable of difference between digitally and standard height measure at distance of 260 cm; d1_L_forearm – variable of difference between digitally and standard left forearm measure at distance of 200 cm, d2_L_forearm – variable of difference between digitally and standard left forearm measure at distance of 230 cm, d3_L_forearm – variable of difference between digitally and standard left forearm measure at distance of 260 cm; d1_L_lower leg – variable of difference between digitally and standard left lower leg measure at distance of 200 cm, d2_L_lower leg – variable of difference between digitally and standard left lower leg measure at distance of 230 cm, d3_L_lower leg – variable of difference between digitally and standard left lower leg measure at distance of 260 cm.

Measurement errors in body dimensions for data collected with Kinect presented in Samejima et al. [24] revealed average error rates for measurement items: height (3.31%), mid-patellar height (6.58%), forearm length (6.68%). It is in line, considering selected methodology and protocol, with our results (Figs. 7, 8, 9 and 10).

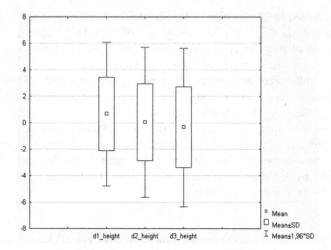

Fig. 7. Differences in descriptive parameters for variable height [12]; ***d1_height*** – *variable of difference between digitally and standard height measure at distance of 200* cm, ***d2_height*** – *variable of difference between digitally and standard height measure at distance of 230* cm, ***d3_height*** – *variable of difference between digitally and standard height measure at distance of 260* cm.

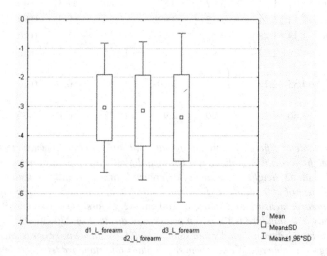

Fig. 8. Differences in descriptive parameters for variable left forearm length [12]; ***d1_L_ forearm*** – *variable of difference between digitally and standard left forearm measure at distance of 200* cm, ***d2_L_forearm*** – *variable of difference between digitally and standard left forearm measure at distance of 230* cm, ***d3_L_forearm*** – *variable of difference between digitally and standard left forearm measure at distance of 260* cm.

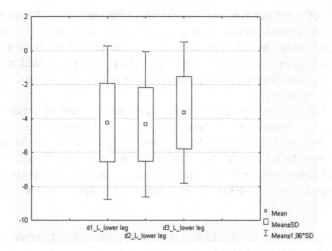

Fig. 9. Differences in descriptive parameters for variable left lower leg length [12]; *d1_L_lower leg* – *variable of difference between digitally and standard left lower leg measure at distance of 200 cm*, *d2_L_ lower leg* – *variable of difference between digitally and standard left lower leg measure at distance of 230 cm*, *d3_L_ lower leg* – *variable of difference between digitally and standard left lower leg measure at distance of 260 cm.*

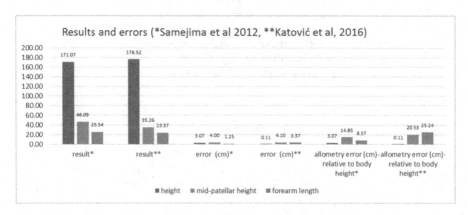

Fig. 10. Comparison of results and mean errors for variables height, left forearm length and left lower leg length between two research – Samejima et al. [24] and Katović et al. [12].

Allometry/proportion error parameter (AEP) represents an error (in cm) that would be detected if mean error of result measured for certain segment (lower leg, i.e. represented with min-patellar height, and forearm length) would be represented on body height. In other words, this parameter AEP reveals weaknesses of instrument regarding precision while measuring body segments based on points mathematically determined for digital protocol. Anatomically determined body points based on bones ensures more precision compared to any other mathematical representation of body points.

Periphery of a subject (i.e. extremities) was measured and calculated with less precision due to several reasons, mostly because of clothes, different measurement standards (IBP/Kinect, in Table 1), imprecise registration of anatomical points etc. Further, differences in representing lower leg length [12] and mid-patellar height [24] were determined by distance from patella to lowest measuring point, i.e. 'knee to ground' vs. 'knee to ankle'.

The correlation matrix between classically and digitally measured variables (Table 5) reveals statistically significant correlation coefficients. It is noticeable that the correlations in variables of *height* and of *left forearm length* decrease proportionally with distance, while in the variable *left lower leg length* increase proportionally with higher distances. Although relatively high, coefficient values of correlations between classically and digitally measured variables are not sufficient for this type of measuring instrument.

Table 5. Correlations between classically and digitally measured body height, left forearm length and left lower leg length [12].

	D1	D2	D3
A_height	0.944	0.940	0.935
A_L_ *forearm*	0.776	0.745	0.614
A_L_ *lower leg*	0.616	0.646	0.664

A_height, A_L_ *forearm* & A_L_ *lower leg* - classically measured *body height*, *left forearm length* and *left lower leg length*, D1 - digitally measured at 200 cm distance, D2 - digitally measured at 230 cm distance, D3 - digitally measured height at 260 cm distance.)

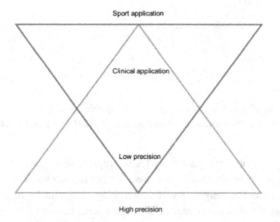

Fig. 11. Clinical/sport application controversy.

Clinical application with high precision demands high reliability due to reductive nature of analysed phenomena. As trend of reducing sport phenomena to controllable and measurable quantitative variables continues and accelerates, demands for high precision and reliability also grows. Notational analysis lowers the scale to kinematics, and biomechanics enter notation analysis. Both clinical and sport application demand diagnostic tools with high reliability and precision, however despite high demands, lower precision tests may find their place in many indirect application, and by the way those may break conservative 'clinical/sport application controversy' represented on Fig. 11.

4 Conclusions

Classical anthropometry based on IBP is precise, but time consuming, kinematics in biomechanical analysis based on classical inverse dynamics are clinically applicable, but assessed with often very expensive instruments and 'limited' laboratory environment, and sport analyses based on notational analysis are not objective and reductive enough.

Main goal of this paper was to test the idea of validation of low cost, time economized, big and relevant data access, user friendly, etc., solution for bridging and evolution in (1) anthropometry - of static/current into dynamic/fluid insight and morphology tracking, (2) biomechanics - of kinematics into VR environments, (3) sport – of construct/hypothetic into convergence of large scale kinematics and low scale notational analysis. Convergence of IBP, inverse dynamic (e.g. Davis) protocols, Kinect SDK's and other approaches to static and dynamic precision and validity, enables more automated, in situ, cheaper and verifiable approach to kinesiological, sport and medicine, phenomena.

Initial findings bring conclusion that digital measurements with Kinect are not appropriate for clinical trials demanding extremely high precision, and that there is no statistical evidence that could differentiate distances of examinee from Kinect sensor in order to define optimal distance. Reliability of Kinect sensor is excellent for height and acceptable for left forearm length and left lower leg length. Small errors occur due to clothing, illumination, sensor height and distance, which is in line with previous research (e.g. Clarkson et al. [4] where results showed that the 3D scanning system 'systematically overestimate volume', Espitia-Contreras et al. [8], etc.)

Acknowledgements. Research was conducted by joint Research Group of Laboratory for Sports Medicine & Exercise - Kinantropometry and Biomechanics Laboratory of the Institute of Kinesiology, Faculty of Kinesiology, as a part of joint IRCRO project "Development of a Computer System for Digital Measurements of the Human Body", between the Faculty of Kinesiology and companies Live Good j.d.o.o. and CITUS d.o.o. Initial conclusions were presented at icSPORTS 2016 in Porto, Portugal [12]. Authors declare that there is no conflict of interest.

References

1. Boonbrahm, P., Sewata, L., Boonbrahm, S.: Transforming 2D human data into 3D model for augmented reality applications. Procedia Comput. Sci. **75**(Vare), 28–33 (2015). https://doi.org/10.1016/j.procs.2015.12.193
2. Cippitelli, E., Gasparrini, S., Spinsante, S., Gambi, E.: Kinect as a tool for gait analysis: validation of a real-time joint extraction algorithm working in side view. Sensors (Basel, Switzerland) **15**(1), 1417–1434 (2015). https://doi.org/10.3390/s150101417
3. Clarkson, S., Wheat, J., Heller, B., Choppin, S.: Assessment of a Microsoft Kinect-based 3D scanning system for taking body segment girth measurements: a comparison to ISAK and ISO standards. J. Sports Sci. **34**(11), 1006–1014 (2016). https://doi.org/10.1080/02640414.2015.1085075
4. Clarkson, S., Wheat, J., Heller, B., Choppin, S.: Assessing the suitability of the Microsoft Kinect for calculating person specific body segment parameters. In: 4th IEEE Workshop on Consumer Depth Cameras for Computer Vision, Zurich, Switzerland, 6 September 2014 (2014)
5. Dell Inc.: Dell Statistica (Data Analysis Software System), Version 12.7 (2016). software. dell.com
6. De Rosario, H., Belda-Lois, J.M., Fos, F., Medina, E., Poveda-Puente, R., Kroll, M.: Correction of joint angles from Kinect for balance exercising and assessment. J. Appl. Biomech. **30**(2), 294–299 (2014). https://doi.org/10.1123/jab.2013-0062
7. Dutta, A., Chugh, S., Banerjee, A., Dutta, A.: Point-of-care-testing of standing posture with Wii balance board and Microsoft Kinect during transcranial direct current stimulation: a feasibility study. NeuroRehabilitation **34**(4), 789–798 (2014). https://doi.org/10.3233/NRE-141077
8. Espitia-Contreras, A., Sanchez-Caiman, P., Uribe-Quevedo, A.: Development of Kinect-Base Anthropometric Measurement Application. Industrial Engineering, Nueva Grenada Mil. University (2015)
9. Galna, B., et al.: Retraining function in people with Parkinson's disease using the Microsoft Kinect: game design and pilot testing. J. NeuroEng. Rehabil. **11**(1), 1–12 (2014). https://doi.org/10.1186/1743-0003-11-60
10. Gao, Z., Yu, Y., Zhou, Y., Du, S.: Leveraging two Kinect sensors for accurate full-body motion capture. Sensors (Switzerland) **15**(9), 24297–24317 (2015). https://doi.org/10.3390/s150924297
11. Gasparrini, S., Cippitelli, E., Spinsante, S., Gambi, E.: A depth-based fall detection system using a Kinect® sensor. Sensors (Basel, Switzerland) **14**(2), 2756–2775 (2014). https://doi.org/10.3390/s140202756
12. Katović, D., et al.: Development of computer system for digital measurement of human body: initial findings. In: Proceedings of the 4th International Congress on Sport Sciences Research and Technology Support, icSPORTS, vol. 1, pp. 147–153 (2016). ISBN 978-989-758-205-9. https://doi.org/10.5220/0006086001470153
13. Lim, D., Kim, C., Jung, H., Jung, D., Chun, K.: Use of the Microsoft Kinect system to characterize balance ability during balance training. Clin. Interv. Aging **10**, 1077–1083 (2015). https://doi.org/10.2147/CIA.S85299
14. Lun, R., Zhao, W.: A survey of applications and human motion recognition with Microsoft Kinect. Int. J. Pattern Recogn. Artif. Intell. **29** (2015). http://doi.org/10.1142/S0218001415550083

15. Mentiplay, B.F., Clark, R.A., Mullins, A., Bryant, A.L., Bartold, S., Paterson, K.: Reliability and validity of the Microsoft Kinect for evaluating static foot posture. J. Foot Ankle Res. **6** (1), 14 (2013). https://doi.org/10.1186/1757-1146-6-14
16. Mišigoj-Duraković, M.: Kinantropologija: biološki aspekti tjelesnog vježbanja. Kineziološki fakultet Sveučilišta u Zagrebu, Zagreb (2008)
17. Mobini, A., Behzadipour, S., Saadat, M.: Test-retest reliability of Kinect's measurements for the evaluation of upper body recovery of stroke patients. Biomed. Eng. Online 1–13 (2015). http://doi.org/10.1186/s12938-015-0070-0
18. Motiian, S., Pergami, P., Guffey, K., Mancinelli, C.A., Doretto, G.: Automated extraction and validation of children's gait parameters with the Kinect. Biomed. Eng. Online **14**(112), 1–36 (2015). https://doi.org/10.1186/s12938-015-0102-9
19. Oh, B.-L., Kim, J., Kim, J., Hwang, J.-M., Lee, J.: Validity and reliability of head posture measurement using Microsoft Kinect. Br. J. Ophthalmol. 1–5 (2014). http://doi.org/10.1136/bjophthalmol-2014-305095
20. Pfister, A., West, A.M., Bronner, S., Noah, J.A.: Comparative abilities of Microsoft Kinect and Vicon 3D motion capture for gait analysis. J. Med. Eng. Technol. **1902**(5), 1–7 (2014). https://doi.org/10.3109/03091902.2014.909540
21. Procházka, A., Vyšata, O., Vališ, M., Ťupa, O., Schätz, M., Mařík, V.: Use of the image and depth sensors of the Microsoft Kinect for the detection of gait disorders. Neural Comput. Appl. **26**(7), 1621–1629 (2015). https://doi.org/10.1007/s00521-015-1827-x
22. Robinson, M., Parkinson, M.B.: Estimating anthropometry with Microsoft Kinect. In: Proceedings of the 2nd International Digital Human Modeling Symposium, May 2013
23. Saenz-de-Urturi, Z., Garcia-Zapirain Soto, B.: Kinect-based virtual game for the elderly that detects incorrect body postures in real time. Sensors **16**(5), 704 (2016). https://doi.org/10.3390/s16050704
24. Samejima, I., Maki, K., Kagami, S., Kouchi, M., Mizoguchi, H.: A body dimensions estimation method of subject from a few measurement items using Kinect. In: Conference Proceedings - IEEE International Conference on Systems, Man and Cybernetics, pp. 3384–3389 (2012). http://doi.org/10.1109/ICSMC.2012.6378315
25. Sevick, M., Eklund, E., Mensch, A., Foreman, M., Standeven, J., Engsberg, J.: Using free internet videogames in upper extremity motor training for children with cerebral palsy. Behav. Sci. **6**(2), 10 (2016). https://doi.org/10.3390/bs6020010
26. Shapi'i, A., Bahari, N.N., Arshad, H., Zin, N.A.M., Mahayuddin, Z.R.: Rehabilitation exercise game model for post-stroke using Microsoft Kinect camera. In: 2015 2nd International Conference on Biomedical Engineering (ICoBE), pp. 1–6, March 2015. http://doi.org/10.1109/ICoBE.2015.7235882
27. Springer, S., Seligmann, G.Y.: Validity of the Kinect for gait assessment: a focused review. Sensors (Switzerland) **16**(2), 1–13 (2016). https://doi.org/10.3390/s16020194
28. Taha, Z., Hassan, M.S.S., Yap, H.J., Yeo, W.K.: Preliminary investigation of an innovative digital motion analysis device for badminton athlete performance evaluation. Procedia Eng. **147**, 461–465 (2016). https://doi.org/10.1016/j.proeng.2016.06.341
29. Xu, H., Yu, Y., Zhou, Y., Li, Y., Du, S.: Measuring accurate body parameters of dressed humans with large-scale motion using a Kinect sensor. Sensors (Basel, Switzerland) **13**(9), 11362–11384 (2013). https://doi.org/10.3390/s130911362
30. Zhang, Y., Zheng, J., Magnenat-Thalmann, N.: Example-guided anthropometric human body modeling. Vis. Comput. **31**(12), 1615–1631 (2015). https://doi.org/10.1007/s00371-014-1043-1

New Approaches in Measuring
to the Calculations and Analysis Modelling
of Breath-by-Breath Alveolar Gas
Exchanges in Humans

C. Capelli$^{(\boxtimes)}$

Department of Physical Performances, Norwegian School of Sport Sciences,
Sognsveien 220, 0806 Oslo, Norway
carlo.capelli@nih.no

Abstract. The pros and cons of different algorithms developed for estimating breath-by-breath (B-by-B) alveolar O_2 transfer ($\dot{V}O_{2A}$) will be detailed and discussed. $\dot{V}O_{2,A}$ is the difference between O_2 uptake at the mouth and changes in alveolar O_2 stores ($\Delta \dot{V}O_{2,si}$), which, for any given breath, are equal to the alveolar volume change at constant $F_{AO_2}[(F_{AiO_2} \times \Delta V_{Ai})]$ plus the O_2 alveolar fraction change at constant alveola volume $[V_{Ai-1} \times (F_{Ai}-F_{Ai-1})_{O_2}]$, where V_{Ai-1} is the alveolar volume at the beginning of a breath. Therefore, $\dot{V}O_{2,A}$ can be determined B-by-B if V_{Ai-1} is: (i) set equal to the subject's FRC (algorithm of Auchincloss, A) or to zero; (ii) measured (optoelectronic plethysmography, OEP); (iii) selected according to a procedure that minimises B-by-B variability (algorithm of Busso and Robbins, BR). Alternatively, the respiratory cycle can be redefined as the time between equal FO_2 in two subsequent breaths (algorithm of Grønlund, G), making any assumption of V_{Ai-1} unnecessary. All the above methods allow an unbiased estimate of $\dot{V}O_{2,A}$ at steady state, albeit with different precision. However, the algorithms "per se" affect the parameters describing the B-by-B kinetics during exercise transitions. Among these approaches, BR and G, by increasing the signal to noise ratio of the measurements, reduce the number of exercise repetitions necessary to study $\dot{V}O_{2,A}$ kinetics, compared to A approach. OEP and G (though technically challenging and conceptually still debated), thanks to their ability to track ΔVO_{2s} changes during the early phase of exercise transitions, appear rather promising for investigating B-by-B gas exchange.

Keywords: Breath by-Breath alveolar gas exchanges · Gas exchange kinetics · Alveolar gas stores · Time constant · End expiratory alveolar volume

1 Introduction

The study of the oxygen uptake ($\dot{V}O_2$) kinetics at the onset of exercise in humans has attracted the interest of exercise physiologists since the groundbreaking investigations of Krogh and Lindhard and Hill and Lupton [19, 20] who first described the mono-exponential increase of $\dot{V}O_2$ at the beginning of a constant work rate (CWR) exercise. In spite of the limited technological tools available at those times, the investigators

© Springer Nature Switzerland AG 2019
J. Cabri et al. (Eds.): icSPORTS 2016/2017, CCIS 975, pp. 100–115, 2019.
https://doi.org/10.1007/978-3-030-14526-2_7

were already able to describe the mono-exponential increase of $\dot{V}O_2$ obtained by imposing this exercise modality. Thanks to their work, and to that of several other investigators who followed, fundamental concepts such as, for instance, the O_2 deficit were developed and they formed the theoretical framework of muscular bioenergetics as we now conceive and explain.

The study of $\dot{V}O_2$ kinetics boosted during the seventies thanks to the development, first of analogical computing systems [21], and later of digital computers interfaced with gas sensors and ventilatory flow transducers. Thanks to these technical improvement, it was possible to describe and show on-line the dynamic response of gas exchange and ventilation with the highest possible time resolution, i.e. Breath-by-Breath (B-by-B) [6, 7].

The data collected thereby have permitted to understand the factors that dictate $\dot{V}O_2$ kinetics at the beginning of exercise of different intensities in a broad variety of conditions and in several categories of subjects. The important physiological meaning of $\dot{V}O_2$ kinetics resides in the fact that it is considered to provide an integrative view of the aerobic metabolism response of the exercising muscles and of the dynamic response of the cardiovascular convective transport of O_2 from the lungs to the periphery. But in order to accept this view, a necessary proviso is required. Namely, we must be confident that the volume of the O_2 measured over a single breath ($VO_{2,Ai}$) strictly corresponds to the volume of gas crossing by diffusion, over the very same interval of time, the alveolar – capillary barrier. Only in this case, the Fick principle applied to O_2 exchange holds true:

$$\dot{V}O_{2,A} = \dot{Q} \times (C_a - C_{\bar{v}})_{O_2} \tag{1}$$

This equations takes into account the physiological causes underpinning the increase of alveolar $\dot{V}O_2$ ($\dot{V}O_{2,A}$) at the exercise onset: the increase of $\dot{Q}$ and the amplification of the artero-venous difference of O_2 due to its progressively increasing extraction of O_2 in the contracting muscles.

Only if this requirement is fully satisfied, we are allowed to investigate how the dynamic response of the cardiovascular system and the rate of muscular oxidative metabolism may modulate $\dot{V}O_{2,A}$ and consider its kinetics as a proxy of the response of O_2 muscular consumption with the possible distorting modulation introduced by $\dot{Q}$ response. On these bases, and taking for granted that we were able to estimate in a reliable and accurate manner B-by-B $\dot{V}O_{2,A}$, a considerable amount of data have been collected by several investigators who tried to establish which were its main determinants during exercise. However, this review is not focused on the physiological factors limiting or dictating $\dot{V}O_{2,A}$ kinetics in humans and on how it can be used to get insightful information on the behaviour of the muscular oxidative metabolism in vivo. To this aim, the reader is kindly referred to recent and extensive reviews on this topic [22, 23]. Rather, we will focus on some crucial methodological aspects. The first one considers that very few studies have been devoted to the investigations of the performances of the various algorithms used to estimate alveolar-capillary gas exchange on a B-by-B basis in terms of signal to noise ratio. Second, we will discuss whether they may substantially affect the statistical estimation of the parameters describing the kinetics. In this regard, we would like to underline that this important methodological detail is sometimes, or even often, overlooked, since it's pretty common to note that several investigations on $\dot{V}O_{2,A}$ kinetics do not specify whether the investigators properly considered the gas exchanges across the membrane or, rather, they analysed the volumes of O_2 transferred at mouth.

2   Breath-by-Breath Gas Exchanges: Premises

To assess the net alveolar-to-capillary gas transfer of over a given breath i, the changes in the amount of gas stored in the lungs have to be taken into account [4]. For instance, the net amount of O_2 (from now on, we will take O_2 as an example for any gas exchanged at the alveolar level) entering the blood over a single breath i ($VO_{2,Ai}$) is given by:

$$VO_{2,Ai} = VO_{2,mi} - \Delta VO_{2,si} \tag{2}$$

where $VO_{2,mi}$ represent the volumes of gas transferred during breath i at the mouth level and $\Delta VO_{2,si}$ is the change of the alveolar O_2 stores occurring in the same breath i.

A simple example will help us understand the impact of alveolar O_2 stores variations on B-by-B assessment of $\dot{V}O_{2,A}$. Let's imagine a subject who performs a very short inspiration. The inspired air is relatively rich in O_2 (about 21% in volume), but the volume of O_2 introduced into the airways during the inspiration of breath i ($VO_{2I,i}$), given by the product of a high F_IO_2 times a small V_I, will be also small. Afterwards, let's imagine that the same subject takes a very long and deep expiration during which he/she exhales a mixture poorer in O_2 ($F_EO_2 \approx 0.16$–0.17, on average). However, since the O_2 fraction is now multiplied by a large V_E, the resulting $VO_{2E,i}$ is large. In this case, the difference $VO_{2I,i} - VO_{2E,I}$, i.e. $VO_{2,mi}$, will be very small or even negative! This is preposterous, because it would imply that the subject, according to the rule of signs used to describe gas exchanges, "produced" rather than "took up" O_2. Of course, this cannot be the case, since the alveolar partial pressure of O_2 (P_AO_2) has not been perturbed, even during this unusual breath, to such an extent to reverse the diffusion of O_2 from the capillaries to the alveoli. The absurd outcome of these calculations directly results from having neglected in the mass-balance equation for $VO_{2,Ai}$ (Eq. 2) the corresponding changes of lung O_2 stores ($\Delta VO_{2,si}$). Indeed, during this odd breath, $\Delta VO_{2,si}$ markedly decreased and the algebraic sum of the large drop of $\Delta VO_{2,si}$ plus the small or negative $VO_{2,mi}$ still yields a positive $VO_{2,Ai}$. Therefore, we should have understood by now what was somehow dogmatically stated in Eq. 2: if we aim to estimate the O_2 alveolar-capillary transfer over a single breath, we must quantify, together with $VO_{2,mi}$, also $\Delta VO_{2,si}$. If we can neglect the fluctuations of $\Delta VO_{2,si}$ over a long series of breath – as we usually do when we measure the O_2 uptake by using mixing chamber systems because $\Delta VO_{2,si}$ usually represents a negligible fraction of the total volume exchanged at the mouth and we average the O_2 uptake over a series of breaths – we can not disregard them if we aim to measure B-by-B $\dot{V}O_{2,A}$. This is of paramount importance when large and sudden changes in $\Delta VO_{2,si}$ likely occur as at beginning of exercise: in this case the differences between $\dot{V}O_{2,m}$ and $\dot{V}O_{2,A}$ may become substantial, as $\dot{V}O_{2,m}$ does not consider $\Delta VO_{2,si}$ [29].

3 Breath-by-Breath Gas Transfer at the Mouth

$VO_{2,mi}$ is the difference between the inspired volume of O_2 ($VO_{2I,i}$) minus the subsequent expired volume ($VO_{2E,i}$):

$$VO_{2,mi} = \int \dot{V}_I \times F_IO_2 dt - \int \dot{V}_E \times F_EO_2 dt \qquad (3)$$

where F_IO_2 and F_EO_2 are the instantaneous O_2 fractions in the inspired (usually set constant and equal to 0.2095) and expired air, respectively, and $\dot{V}_I$ and $\dot{V}_E$ (both reduced to STPD conditions) are the instantaneous inspiratory and expiratory flow. The product of F_IO_2 times $\dot{V}_I$ and of F_EO_2 times $\dot{V}_E$ are integrated over the corresponding phases of the respiratory cycle and the latter is subtracted from the former to obtain $VO_{2,mi}$. In some instances, $\dot{V}_I$ is calculated from the measured $\dot{V}_E$ by applying the so-called Haldane transformation based on the realistic assumption that the net N_2 transfer across the alveolar membrane ($\dot{V}N_{2,Ai}$) is nil:

$$VN_{2,Ai} = VN_{2,mi} - \Delta VN_{2,si} = 0 \qquad (4)$$

Since only over several consecutive breaths (i.e. >5) the algebraic sum of the changes in alveolar nitrogen stores, $\Delta VN_{2,si}$, can be legitimately considered equal to 0, and hence ignored in the N_2 mass-balance Eq. 4, $VN_{2,Ai} = 0$ is actually equal to the difference of $VN_{2I,i}$ minus $VN_{2E,i}$ only if we consider a series of breaths. Only in this case, therefore, we can then calculate V_I (or $\dot{V}_I$) by knowing F_IN_2 (set constant and equal to 0.7903) and by measuring V_E (or $\dot{V}_E$) and F_EN_2 as:

$$V_I = V_E \times \frac{F_EN_2}{F_IN_2} \qquad (5)$$

Therefore, the Haldane transformation, which is classically utilised in the standard open circuit method with Douglas bags and in the systems based on the utilisation of mixing chambers, cannot be by any means used to calculate V_I from measured V_E over a single breath, because the requirement of $\Delta VN_{2,si}$ equal to 0 does not hold true. However, even when the $VO_{2,mi}$ is calculated using direct measures of V_I and V_E and of the gas fractions, the calculation of B-by-B $VO_{2,mi}$ is prone to yield values that can be substantially different from $VO_{2,Ai}$, especially when large and sudden changes in $\Delta VO_{2,si}$ are likely to occur as, for instance, at beginning of CWR exercise (see paragraphs below).

4 Quantification of Alveolar O_2 Changes and Breath-by-Breath Alveolar Gas Transfer

As it has been already outlined, B-by-b $\dot{V}O_{2,A}$ kinetics can be used to obtain insightful information on the mechanisms coupling muscular O_2 utilisation rate to the dynamics of ventilatory and cardiovascular convective transport of O_2. However, in order to estimate the alveolar-to-capillary transfer of O_2 in a single breath - $VO_{2,Ai}$ -, we have understood that we need to quantify, in parallel with $VO_{2,mi}$, the corresponding $\Delta VO_{2,si}$.

Auchincloss was the first to propose an algorithm (referred to hereafter as A) incorporating $\Delta VO_{2,si}$ in the calculation of B-by-B at the alveolar level [4]. $\Delta VO_{2,si}$ occurring in breath i is given by:

$$\Delta VO_{2,si} = V_{Ai-1} \times (F_{Ai} - F_{Ai-1})_{O_2} + FA_{iO_2} \times \Delta V_{Ai} \tag{6}$$

where V_{Ai-1} is the end-expiratory alveolar volume before the beginning of breath i, F_{Ai} and FA_{i-1} are the O_2 alveolar fractions in the current (i) and previous ($i - 1$) breaths, and ΔV_{Ai} is the alveolar volume change measured as the difference between V_{Ai} and V_{Ai-1}, both assessed at the end of two subsequent expirations. The first term on the right-hand side of Eq. 6 accounts for the changes in $\Delta VO_{2,si}$ due to the gas fraction changes occurring at a constant alveolar volume; the second term is due to the changes in alveolar volume at a constant alveolar gas fraction. Among the variables appearing in Eq. 6, ΔV_{Ai} can be calculated B-by-B by assuming a net $VN_{2,Ai}$ equal to 0 (a reasonable assumption holding even over a single breath, provided that we consider the corresponding alveolar N_2 store variation, $VN_{2,si}$ and measure the N_2 exchanged at the mouth, $VN_{2,mi}$) [4, 26]:

$$VN_{2,Ai} = VN_{2,mi} - VN_{2,si} = 0 \tag{7}$$

In fact, by substituting in Eq. 4 the expression for $VN_{2,si}$ obtained from the right-hand side of Eq. 6 as applied now to N_2, we obtain, after rearranging:

$$\Delta V_{Ai} = [VN_{2,mi} - V_{Ai-1} \times (F_{Ai} - F_{Ai-1})_{N_2}]/F_{AN_2} \tag{8}$$

Once ΔV_{Ai} has been calculated, it can be utilised in Eq. 6 to obtain $\Delta VO_{2,si}$, which, in turn, is needed for calculating $VO_{2,Ai}$ (Eq. 2). $\dot{V}O_{2,Ai}$ can then be finally obtained by dividing ΔV_{Ai} by the duration (Δt) of the corresponding breathing cycle.

Giezendanner et al. [15] proposed an alternative approach to the calculation of ΔV_{Ai} as the difference between V_{Ii} and V_{Ei}, claiming that this procedure introduces, for $0.83 < RR < 1.3$, a maximal error of less than 1.4%. Even though appealing for its simplicity, this approach is conceptually questionable. Let us suppose, for instance, that starting from a given V_A, a subject inhales a certain volume of air (Fig. 1) without reaching vital capacity (VC); he/she then exhales, but does not attain functional residual capacity (FRC). The difference ΔV_{Ai} can be calculated as $V_{Ii} - V_{Ei}$ only and only if the amount of O_2 transferred from the alveoli to the capillary is identical to the volume of CO_2 added to the alveolar gas over the same respiratory cycle, a fact that is strictly true only if RR is 1.

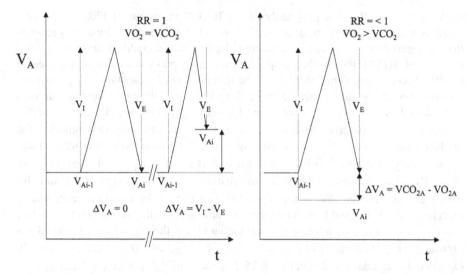

Fig. 1. Alveolar volume as a function of time. The left panel refers to two breaths during which gas exchanges occur, with a RR maintained equal to the unit. In the first breath, V_I is identical to V_E, hence ΔV_A is equal to zero. In the second, V_I is larger to V_E, but ΔV_A can be still calculated as the difference $V_I - V_E$ as the volume of O_2 taken up by the alveoli is identical to that of CO_2 added during the same breath, and V_{A1-1} is unchanged. The right panel refers to a RR < 1 and the hypothesis that $V_I = V_E$. In this case, even if the inspired and expired volumes are identical, ΔV_A cannot be calculated from their difference as ΔV_A is given by $VCO_{2A} - VO_{2A}$. In turn, these two quantities can be calculated only if ΔVO_{2s} and ΔVCO_{2s} are known. As ΔV_A is one of the components of the two latter entities, we are trapped in a circular argument and must estimate ΔV_A by using an independent alternative approach (From Capelli et al. [10]).

If we assume that end-tidal gas fractions are reasonable estimates of alveolar gas fractions, the only quantity not directly measurable on a B-by-B basis in Eqs. 6 and 8 remains V_{Ai-1}. This must therefore be given a predetermined value. To this aim, Auchincloss et al. [4] assumed V_{Ai-1} to be equal to the FRC of the subject. The original approach proposed by Auchincloss was later modified and implemented for practical purposes by Beaver and colleagues [7] and has since then been extensively applied in the study of $\dot{V}O_{2,A}$ kinetics.

The A algorithm was extensively tested by di Prampero and Lafortuna [14] who showed that all nominal V_{Ai-1} values taken to estimate steady-state $\dot{V}O_{2,A}$ yield the same average and greatly reduce B-by-B variability with respect to $\dot{V}O_{2,m}$. Moreover, the magnitude of B-by-B $\dot{V}O_{2,A}$ noise strictly depends on the absolute value of the nominal V_{Ai-1} used for calculations. Finally, the authors underlined that the assumption of V_{Ai-1} equal to a constant FRC is not justified, since end-expiratory lung volume undergoes a sudden drop at the onset of CWR exercise and fluctuates around an average value once steady state has been attained, as subsequently shown [2, 26, 29].

To circumvent some of the drawbacks inherent to A, other "Auchincloss-derived" algorithms have been proposed and tested.

Wessel and colleagues [26] analysed the B-by-B variations of FRC during tidal ventilation and their effect on measured O_2 and CO_2 gas exchanges. First, they showed that FRC undergoes a substantial absolute B-by-B variation within a range from +360 to −360 ml (BTPS), thus further invalidating the assumption of a constant V_{Ai-1} equal to FRC. Second, they demonstrated that the introduction of a constant V_{Ai-1} generates a larger imprecision in the calculation of B-by-B $\Delta VO_{2,si}$ the one potentially derived from directly measuring the difference $(F_{Ai} - F_{Ai-1})_{O_2}$ (see Eq. 6). Hence, in the proposed method (referred to hereafter as W), the authors suggested ignoring the product $V_{Ai-1} \times (F_{Ai} - F_{Ai-1})_{O_2}$ appearing in Eq. 6, because the former term cannot be accurately determined B-by-B and because $(F_{Ai} - F_{Ai-1})_{O_2}$, and even more so $(F_{Ai} - F_{Ai-1})_{CO_2}$, values are negligible (oscillating around an average of ±1 mm Hg) during tidal ventilation. Yet, such is not the case during the transition from rest to exercise. di Prampero and Lafortuna were later able to show that neglecting the product $V_{Ai-1} \times (F_{Ai} - F_{Ai-1})_{O_2}$ introduces a substantial bias in the assessment of B-by-B gas exchanges [14]. As a matter of fact, for a $(F_{Ai} - F_{Ai-1})_{O_2}$ of 0.001, a value commonly exceeded during tidal ventilation [6, 14, 15, 26], the term $V_{Ai-1} \times (F_{Ai} - F_{Ai-1})_{O_2}$ may generate a correction in $\dot{V}O_{2,A}$ of about 50 ml min^{-1} (20–25% of the mean value at rest), for a value of $V_{Ai-1} = 3.5$ l (BTPS). During transients, the weight of this correction may reasonably be even greater to an extent that cannot be neglected.

Swanson [24] proposed an alternative approach (referred to hereafter as S) to circumvent the problems arising from the need to calculate B-by-B $\Delta VO_{2,si}$. He attributed the larger cause of B-by-B $\dot{V}O_{2,A}$ variation to consensual B-by-B variability in $\Delta VO_{2,si}$. By this reasoning, the method that yields the smallest variability of B-by-B $\dot{V}O_{2,A}$ would also yield the most reliable estimate of B-by-B alveolar gas exchanges. Therefore, Swanson proposed considering V_{Ai-1} as equal to the lung volume for which the B-by-B variability in $\dot{V}O_{2,A}$, calculated *a posteriori* over a long series of breaths, is minimised. This he defined as the Effective Lung Volume (ELV), i.e. the end-expiratory lung volume that actually participates in alveolar gas exchanges. When applied during rest-to-exercise transients, this approach assumes, *a priori*, a deterministic variation in ELV as a function of time, an obviously arbitrary hypothesis.

More recently, Busso and Robbins [8] devised a method (referred to hereafter as BR) that implicitly assumes that the "best" method would minimise $\dot{V}O_{2,A}$ variability. In addition, they proposed that the true value of $(F_{Ai} - F_{Ai-1})_{O_2}$ should lie between 0 and $(F_{Ai} - F_{Ai-1})_{O_2}$. This is tantamount to assume that the true value of $\dot{V}O_{2,A}$ is included within those calculated by applying the A and W algorithms, respectively. As a consequence, the retained $\dot{V}O_{2,A}$ values were estimated by minimising their B-by-B variation, subject to the constraint that the final value of $\dot{V}O_{2,A}$ must lie between the values calculated by the A and W algorithms. Busso and Robbins tested their method using a nine-compartment [27], nonhomogeneous, steadily perfused and tidally ventilated lung model, with a realistic breathing pattern. The model simulated a series of $\dot{V}O_{2,A}$ and $\dot{V}CO_{2,A}$ values, wherein the B-by-B variability in the alveolar gas exchanges was due only to variation in the breathing pattern, since O_2 and CO_2 circulatory inflow to the lung model was assumed to be constant. They then showed that their algorithm minimised the model's B-by-B gas exchange variation and assumed therefore that, when applied under realistic conditions, it should yield "true" alveolar gas transfer values.

It has been clearly shown that, in the A algorithm, the only not measurable term in the calculations for estimating lung gas store variations is V_{Ai-1} and that its absolute value directly influences the variability in B-by-B $\dot{V}O_{2,A}$. As illustrated above, although several methods have been proposed to overcome these drawbacks, none of them has introduced the direct measurement of V_{Ai-1}. This problem has been approached thanks to a recently developed technique.

Optoelectronic plethysmography (OEP), a modified motion analysis method, allows the measurement of changes in chest wall volume during breathing [11] by combining chest wall volume changes with preliminary measurements of vital VC and FRC. This makes it possible to accurately determine absolute lung volumes at any point during the breathing cycle and to track the corresponding B-by-B changes of V_{Ai-1} [13]. By combining OEP with assessment of $\dot{V}O_{2,m}$, this technique can be utilised to measure B-by-B $\Delta VO_{2,si}$ and, therefore, B-by-B $VO_{2,Ai}$. Aliverti and colleagues [2] demonstrated that V_{Ai-1} systematically changes at the onset of exercise and of recovery phases, confirming that systematic errors in the calculation of lung gas stores and alveolar gas exchanges are introduced if V_{Ai-1} is assumed to remain constant or to follow a predetermined time course. Furthermore, by using the directly measured B-by-B absolute values of V_{Ai-1}, they calculated B-by-B $\Delta VO_{2,si}$ in steady-state (rest and exercise) and during rest-to-exercise transitions obtaining reliable measures of $\dot{V}O_{2,A}$ and $\dot{V}CO_{2,A}$. Although a method based on the use of OEP, along with standard measures of respiratory gas fractions and flow at the mouth, appears highly promising for research and clinical applications [25], it remains rather time-consuming and technically demanding. At its current stage of technical development, it cannot provide the user with immediate results.

To circumvent the problems inherent in assuming a given value of, or in measuring V_{Ai-1}, other investigators proposed a radically different approach. Grønlund [18] defined the respiratory cycle as the period of time elapsing between equal expiratory FO_2 values, occurring at t_1 and t_2, respectively, in two successive breaths (Fig. 2). Since $FO_{2,t1}$ is identical to $FO_{2,t2}$, the term $V_{Ai-1}(F_{Ai} - F_{Ai-1})_{O_2}$ becomes 0 and, hence, the assumption of a value for V_{Ai-1} becomes unnecessary. Thus, according to Grønlund, the algorithm (referred to hereafter as G) permitting the calculation of $\dot{V}O_{2,A}$ over the interval t_1-t_2 reduces to:

$$VO_{2,A} = \int_{t_2}^{t_1} \dot{V}FO_2 dt - FO_{2t_1}\Delta V_A \qquad (9)$$

where $\dot{V}$ is the respiratory flow, whose sign depends on the phase (inspiration or expiration) considered, FO_{2t1} is the O_2 fraction at time t_1, and ΔV_A the lung volume change over the interval $t_2-t_1 = \Delta t$. The definite integral in Eq. 9 yields the volume of gas exchanged at the mouth over Δt. ΔV_A is obtained from the N_2 balance equation as follows. Having determined the N_2 fraction at t_1 (FN_{2t1}), a time t_3 is identified in the

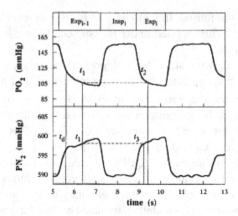

Fig. 2. Recordings of PO_2 and PN_2 during steady-state exercise at 120 W. t_d denotes the time after which the dead space gas had been expired; $Insp_i$ and Exp_i the inspiration and expiration phases of breath i, respectively; and Exp_{i-1} the preceding expiration. Time t_1 is chosen according to specific criteria (see text), times t_2 and t_3 are chosen to yield PO_2 and PN_2 values, respectively, which are identical to those at t_1 (from Capelli et al. [10]).

next breath for which $FN_{2t1} = FN_{2t3}$ (Fig. 2). The alveolar volume change occurring over t1–t3, as given by Eq. 8, then reduces to $\Delta V_A = VN_{2,m}/FN_{2t1}$, where $VN_{2,m}$ is the N_2 exchanged at the mouth between t_1 and t_3 and FN_{2t1} is the N_2 fraction at t_1. Should t_3 not coincide with t_2, the changes in lung volume occurring from t_2 to t_3 must be taken into account. In this respect, it can be assumed that the algebraic sum of the CO_2 and O_2 volumes transferred from t_2 to t_3 is negligible, and ΔV_A occurring over this interval is obtained by integrating $\dot{V}_E$ from t_2 to t_3 ($\int_{t_2}^{t_3} \dot{V}_E dt$). This makes it possible to calculate ΔV_A and to obtain $VO_{2,A}$ over Δt. Finally, $\dot{V}O_{2,A}$ is given by the ratio of $VO_{,2A}$ to Δt. The algorithms described above apply to alveolar O_2 transfer. Simple modifications make it also possible to obtain alveolar CO_2 transfer.

The G algorithm has been extensively tested to measure B-by-B alveolar gas exchanges at rest and during exercise at steady state. First, the method was demonstrated accurate, compared to the standard open circuit in measuring $\dot{V}O_{2,A}$ and $\dot{V}CO_{2,A}$. Moreover, compared to A and derived algorithms, it increases the signal-to-noise ratio of B-by-B alveolar gas exchanges during moderate intensity exercise at steady state from about 21% with A to 13% with G (Table 1).

An extensive analysis of the residuals obtained from the A and G algorithms was also performed to verify whether their variability could be assimilated to a so-called "white noise" [9]. The residuals were normally distributed, with a mean value of 0. In algorithm A, however, the contiguous values were correlated negatively, showing that the correction for lung gas store changes was alternatively too large or too small, thus making the calculated B-by-B variability in gas alveolar transfer artificially large. The necessity of assuming a given value of V_{Ai-1} has a considerable role in the generation of this variability, since it is a multiplier for the difference $(F_{Ai} - F_{Ai-1})_{O_2}$. The latter

Table 1. Mean, SD and CV of $\dot{V}O_{2,A}$ and $\dot{V}CO_{2,A}$ values at steady state obtained in a subjects pedalling during submaximal intensity exercise at 60 W together with the corresponding values measured at the mouth (modified form Capelli et al. [9]).

	Mouth	Auchincloss	Wessel	Swanson	Busso - Robbins	Grønlund
$\dot{V}O_{2,A}$						
$\bar{x}$ (L min^{-1})	1.359	1.123	1.129	1.391	1.128	1.139
SD (L min^{-1})	0.329	0.239	0.137	0.129	0.134	0.152
CV (%)	24.2	21.3	12.1	9.3	11.9	13.3
$\dot{V}CO_{2,A}$						
$\bar{x}$ (L min^{-1})	1.144	1.34	1.129	1.129	1.396	1.402
SD (L min^{-1})	0.134	0.288	0.137	0.137	0.100	0.186
CV (%)	11.7	20.6	12.1	12.1	7.1	13.3

may be positive or negative depending on the difference between the alveolar ventilation of two subsequent breaths. Hence, the term $V_{Ai-1} \times (F_{Ai} - F_{Ai-1})_{O_2}$ may be subtracted or added in Eq. 3, its amplitude depending on the assumed value of V_{Ai-1}.

The main drawback of the G algorithm is the fact that B-by-B gas exchange values can be calculated only during off-line analysis of gas fractions and respiratory flow signals, as the method seeks equal expiratory FO_2 values occurring in two successive, but not necessarily adjacent, breaths.

5 Impact of Using the Various Algorithms for Computing B-by-B $\dot{V}O_{2,A}$ on the Parameters that Describe the Dynamic Characteristics of $\dot{V}O_{2,A}$ Kinetic

This paragraph will specifically address the impact of using various algorithms for computing B-by-B $\dot{V}O_{2,A}$ on the parameters that describe its kinetics.

As already outlined, the response of $\dot{V}O_{2,A}$ at the beginning of CWR exercise performed at moderate intensity, i.e. below the lactate threshold (LT) or gas exchange threshold (GET), is characterized by a rise that is modelled as a bi-exponential increasing function [22]. The first component - phase I, or cardiodynamic phase - is followed by the second component - phase II or primary phase – until the oxygen uptake at steady state ($\dot{V}O_{2,ss}$) is attained. $\dot{V}O_{2,A}$ increase in phase II is considerably slower than the one observed during phase I, as its time constant τ_2 is about 20 s in young, healthy, trained subjects [22]. The kinetics of phase 1 have been related to the delay and amplitude of the cardiodynamic response to exercise onset [28], whereas τ_2 has been considered to describe the rate of adjustment of muscle VO_2 during metabolic transitions [17]. As such, the correct estimation of $\dot{V}O_{2,A}$ is, again, of paramount importance to avoid temporal distortions of the signal and therefore misinterpretation of the underlying physiology.

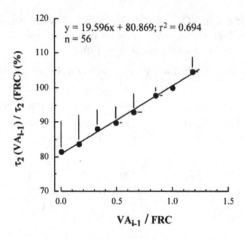

Fig. 3. Mean differences between the time constants of Phase II of oxygen uptake kinetics (τ_2) obtained with the A algorithm, at different values for V_{Ai-1}, and that estimated from the G algorithm (normalised to the values obtained by using algorithm G and expressed as percentages) plotted as a function of the corresponding mean ratios of V_{Ai-1} to FRC (from Cautero et al. [12]). When assuming $V_{Ai-1} = 0$ (i.e., algorithm W), τ_2 was about 7% longer (36.6 s vs. 34.3 s) ($P < 0.05$) than that estimated according to algorithm G. When V_{Ai-1} was set equal to FRC, the difference increased to 31% (i.e., 45.0 s vs. 34.3 s), indicating that the absolute value of V_{Ai-1} utilised in algorithm A has a large effect on the estimated τ_2 value (From Cautero et al. [12]).

di Prampero and Lafortuna demonstrated that the use of A in the study of $\dot{V}O_{2,A}$ kinetics introduced a substantial uncertainty in the time delay of phase I [14]. More recently, Cautero et al. [12] compared the G and A algorithms, applied to the same signals, by analysing $\dot{V}O_{2,A}$ kinetics at the onset of moderate-intensity, step cycling exercise. Compared to algorithm G, the τ_2 values obtained with algorithm A were systematically larger (Fig. 3) and turned out to be correlated with the V_{Ai-1} values used in the calculations (Fig. 4). The reason why the assumed value of V_{Ai-1} brings about a distortion in the $\dot{V}O_{2,A}$ kinetics (i.e. a proportional increase in τ_2) is that it amplifies the contribution of $(F_{Ai} - F_{Ai-1})_{O_2}$ and $(F_{Ai} - F_{Ai-1})_{N_2}$ to the calculated $\dot{V}O_{2,A}$ value [12]. To better elucidate this concept, first Eqs. 6 and 8 can be combined so that $\Delta VO_{2,s}$ can be expressed as follows:

$$\Delta VO_{2,si} = V_{Ai-1}(F_{Ai} - F_{Ai-1})_{O_2} - \frac{FO_{2,Ai}}{FN_{2,Ai}} V_{Ai-1}(F_{Ai} - F_{Ai-1})_{N_2} + \frac{FO_{2,Ai}}{FN_{2,Ai}} VN_{2,mi} \quad (10)$$

In turn, $VO_{2,Ai}$ is given by:

$$VO_{2,Ai} = VO_{2,mi} - V_{Ai-1}(F_{Ai} - F_{Ai-1})_{O_2} - \frac{FO_{2Ai}}{FN_{2Ai}} V_{Ai-1}$$

$$(F_{Ai} - F_{Ai-1})_{N_2} + \frac{FO_{2,Ai}}{FN_{2,Ai}} VN_{2,mi} \quad (11)$$

At exercise onset, the B-by-B differences in end-tidal O_2 and end-tidal $N_2 \left[(F_{Ai} - F_{Ai-1})_{O_2}, (F_{Ai} - F_{Ai-1})_{N_2} \right]$ respectively decrease and increase for about 50 s, attaining a steady level within about 120 s. Therefore, in this early phase of the transient, they are neither 0 nor can they be assimilated to a random time series. On the contrary, they show a deterministic time course (Fig. 5) that progressively fades into a random one. This implies that the deterministic courses of the two quantities introduce a linear distortion (and therefore a slowing of τ_2), whose role is amplified by the absolute value of V_{Ai-1}.

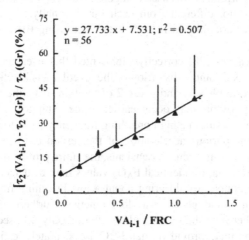

Fig. 4. The time constant of Phase II of oxygen uptake kinetics (τ_2) obtained with the A algorithm using different values for V_{Ai-1}, divided by the value obtained by setting V_{Ai-1} = FRC and expressed as a percentage is plotted as a function of the normalised ratios of V_{Ai-1} to FRC. τ_2 significantly increases with V_{Ai-1} (from Cautero et al. [12]). Indeed, in the range of the V_{Ai-1} values usually assumed in the literature (from 0 [26] to FRC or slightly above [4, 24]), τ_2 varied by about 22% increasing from 36.6 s for V_{Ai-1} = 0 to 45.0 s for V_{Ai-1} = FRC and to 46.8 s for V_{Ai-1} = FRC + 0.5 l (about 125% FRC) (from Cautero et al. [12]).

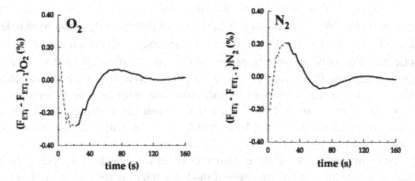

Fig. 5. Breath-to-breath differences in the end-tidal fraction of O_2 expressed in percentages (upper panel, (%)) and nitrogen (lower panel, (%)) after exercise onset. Dotted lines refer to data occurring in Phase I of the transition. See text for more details (from Cautero et al. [12]).

Also the BR algorithm has been applied to analyse $\dot{V}O_{2,A}$ kinetics during constant-load exercise transition of moderate and heavy intensity [16]. The parameters describing $\dot{V}O_{2,A}$ kinetics (time delays, time constants, and amplitudes of primary and slow components of $\dot{V}O_{2,A}$ kinetics) were estimated from B-by-B $\dot{V}O_{2,m}$ and from $\dot{V}O_{2,A}$ calculated by means of the BR, A and W algorithms. The results suggested, in accordance with other authors, that the A algorithm may yield biased estimates of the parameters describing the exponential time course of $\dot{V}O_{2,A}$ at exercise onset. Indeed, significant differences in amplitude, time delay and time constant of the primary phase were shown when algorithm A was used compared with W, $\dot{V}O_{2,m}$ and BR approaches, which, in turn, were not different from each other. Finally, the study confirmed a substantially reduced variability in B-by-B data when using BR compared with algorithm A.

Whipp and colleagues [28] correctly highlighted that even the G approach may theoretically lead to a substantial distortion of the alveolar gas kinetics. Since the slope of F_AO_2 increase during phase 1 and phase 2 of the transients, the value of F_AO_2 that satisfies the required criteria, may occur earlier in the expiratory phase of the subsequent breath. This may result in a high breathing frequency - due to a very short breath - and contribute to a spurious acceleration of the response. Conversely, should the subject hyperventilate during exercise transients, the entire profile of expired F_AO_2 may increase to such a level that no identical F_AO_2 values may be detected in two adjacent expirations. This, of course, would bring about a low breathing frequency – due to a spurious long breath – and generate a slow kinetics. Furthermore, concerning the crucial comparison between the G method and the broadly diffused A algorithm, the above authors claim that, provided that FRC is accurately estimated or directly determined (not forgetting also the potential effect of gravity and of posture), the error in estimating τ_2 with A is substantially reduced in comparison with the value obtained by using G.

We have already underlined that the G algorithm and the OEP approaches overcome the main difficulties inherent with the assessment of B-by-B variation in lung gas stores by either making any assumption of end-alveolar volume unnecessary (the former) or by measuring it directly (the latter).

By applying OEP to B-by-B gas exchange analysis, and thus directly assessing changes in $\Delta VO_{2s,}$ Wüst and colleagues [29] showed that the $\dot{V}O_{2,m}$ data were indeed significantly lower than the $\dot{V}O_{2,A}$ values in the first 15 s of on-transient of step exercise transitions (the opposite being true in the early off-phase, when $\dot{V}O_{2,m}$ values were higher than the $\dot{V}O_{2,A}$ values). This discrepancy was mainly ascribed to a change in pulmonary O_2 stores as assessed by measuring the absolute B-by-B variations in lung volume. Thus, these data once again showed that gas exchange kinetics at the early stage of exercise transient can be accurately described only if ΔVO_{2s} is estimated or directly measured.

G algorithm and the OEP have been utilised to measure B-by-B $\dot{V}O_{2,A}$ during constant-load cycling exercise transients of moderate intensity (60, 90 and 120 W) [3]. Compared to the other methods, the G algorithm had the smallest B-by-B variability. The mean response time (MRT) calculated by using OEP B-by-B data was systematically shorter than by using G (Fig. 6) due to a smaller τ_2 and a larger amplitude of the so-called cardiodynamic phase.

The authors document a sudden decrease in end-expiratory lung volume at exercise onset, due to expiratory muscle activation [1], that is responsible for a prompt reduction in ΔVO_{2s} [29]. Therefore, only OEP would allow an accurate estimate of B-by-B $\dot{V}O_{2,A}$ during the first 30 s of exercise, so carefully tracking the actual amplitude of the cardiodynamic component.

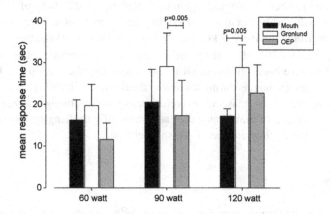

Fig. 6. Mean response time (MRT) values ± standard deviations of $\dot{V}O_2$ kinetics at the three indicated workloads. These were calculated from normalised amplitudes, time delays and time constants estimated by fitting the B-by-B $\dot{V}O_{2m}$ and $\dot{V}O_{2A}$ data calculated with OEP and the G algorithm. The short segments shown above the histograms connect the MRT values that were significantly different. P-values are also indicated (from Aliverti et al. [3]).

Furthermore, the authors speculated that G may be affected by an unknown bias in respect to OEP [3]. Since G omits the term that accounts for the variations in $\Delta VO_{2,s}$ due to gas fraction changes at a constant alveolar volume, it may overlook one of the two sources of ΔVO_{2s}. This potentially weakens the impact of the sudden changes of $\Delta VO_{2,s}$ and therefore may lead to an underestimation of B-by-B $\dot{V}O_{2A}$ in the early phase of the transient.

6 Conclusions

B-by-B gas exchange determination has gained wide acceptance in clinical and physiological applications, despite the fact that there is currently no easy way to reliably measure alveolar-capillary gas transfer.

The main difficulty with the determination of B-by-B alveolar gas exchanges resides in reliable assessment of B-by-B lung gas store variations. To this aim, the knowledge of end-expiratory alveolar volume is required, which, however, cannot be easily measured on a B-by-B basis and so is customarily assumed in the algorithm proposed by Auchincloss [4] and implemented by Beaver [7]. Several recent studies have proposed and evaluated methods that: (i) substantially reduced the noise associated with A algorithm [8, 16], (ii) directly measured B-by-B lung and O_2 store variations (OEP), or (iii) made any assumption regarding the value of the end-expiratory alveolar volume unnecessary (G).

The more commonly applied algorithms yield an unbiased estimate of alveolar O_2 uptake and CO_2 output at steady state. Furthermore, compared to measures at the mouth, all algorithms (and specially so BR and G) cut down the noise-to-signal ratio, so reducing the number of exercise repetitions required for the study of VO_2 kinetics.

Yet, along with this practical advantage, the algorithms "per se" seems to affect the parameters describing the B-by-B kinetics during exercise transitions, making the study of $\dot{V}O_{2A}$ and $\dot{V}CO_{2A}$ B-by-B kinetics during exercise somewhat elusive. Among the approaches that have been reviewed, OEP and G appear rather promising for investigating B-by-B gas exchange during exercise, thanks to their ability to track ΔVO_{2s} changes during the early phase of exercise transitions. Although appealing, these approaches are not free of drawbacks, they are technically challenging and some of the assumptions on which they are based are still debated.

References

1. Aliverti, A., et al.: Human respiratory muscle actions and control during exercise. J. Appl. Physiol. **83**, 1256–1269 (1997)
2. Aliverti, A., Kayser, B., Macklem, P.T.: Breath-by-breath assessment of alveolar gas stores and exchange. J. Appl. Physiol. **96**, 1464–1469 (2004)
3. Aliverti, A., Kaiser, B., Cautero, M., Dellacà, R.L., di Prampero, P.E., Capelli, C.: Pulmonary O_2 kinetics at the onset of exercise is faster when actual changes in alveolar $\dot{V} O_2$ stores are considered. Resp. Physiol. Neurobiol. **1698**, 78–82 (2009)
4. Auchincloss Jr, J.H., Gilbert, R., Baule, G.H.: Effect of ventilation on oxygen transfer during early exercise. J. Appl. Physiol. **21**, 810–818 (1966)
5. Beaver, W.L., Wassermann, K.: Transients in ventilation at start and end of exercise. J. Appl. Physiol. **21**, 390–399 (1968)
6. Beaver, W.L., Wassermann, K., Whipp, B.J.: On-line computer analysis and breath-by-breath graphical display of exercise function test. J. Appl. Physiol. **34**, 128–132 (1973)
7. Beaver, W.L., Lamarra, N., Wasserman, K.: Breath-by-breath measurement of true alveolar gas exchange. J. Appl. Physiol. **51**, 1662–1675 (1981)
8. Busso, T., Robbins, P.A.: Evaluation of estimates of alveolar gas exchange by using a tidally ventilated non-homogenous lung model. J. Appl. Physiol. **82**, 1963–1971 (1997)
9. Capelli, C., Cautero, M., di Prampero, P.E.: New perspectives in breath-by-breath determination of alveolar gas exchanges in humans. Pflügers Arch. **441**, 566–577 (2001)
10. Capelli, C., Cautero, M., Poglgahi, S.: Algorithms, modelling and $\dot{V}O2$ kinetics. Eur. J. Appl. Physiol. **111**, 331–342 (2011)
11. Cala, S.J., et al.: Chest wall and lung volume estimation by optical reflectance motion analysis. J. Appl. Physiol. **81**, 2680–2689 (1996)
12. Cautero, M., Beltrami, A.P., Capelli, C., di Prampero, P.E.: Breath-by-breath alveolar oxygen transfer at the onset of step exercise in humans: methodological implications. Eur. J. Physiol. **88**, 203–231 (2002)

13. Dellacà, R., Aliverti, A., Pelosi, P., Carlesso, E., Chiumello, D., Pedotti, A.: Estimation of end-expiratory variations by optoelectronic plethysmography (OEP). Crit. Care Med. **29**, 1807–1811 (2001)
14. di Prampero, P.E., Lafortuna, C.L.: Breath-by-breath estimate of alveolar gas transfer variability in man at rest and during exercise. J. Physiol. (Lond.) **415**, 459–475 (1989)
15. Giezendanner, D., Cerretelli, P., di Prampero, P.E.: Breath-by-breath alveolar gas exchange. J. Appl. Physiol. **55**, 583–590 (1983)
16. Gimenez, P., Busso, T.: Implications of breath-by-breath oxygen uptake determination on kinetics assessment during exercise. Respir. Physiol. Neurobiol. **162**, 238–241 (2008)
17. Grassi, B., Poole, D.C., Richardson, R.S., Knight, D.R., Erickson, B.K., Wagner, P.D.: Muscle O_2 uptake kinetics in humans: implications for metabolic control. J. Appl. Physiol. **80**, 988–998 (1996)
18. Grønlund, L.: A new method for breath-to-breath determination of oxygen flux across the alveolar membrane. Eur. J. Appl. Physiol. **52**, 167–172 (1984)
19. Hill, A.V., Lupton, H.: Muscular exercise, lactic acid, and the supply and utilization of oxygen. Q. J. Med. **16**, 135–171 (1923)
20. Krogh, A., Lindhard, J.: The regulation of respiration and circulation during the initial stages of muscular work. J. Physiol. (Lond.) **47**, 112–136 (1913)
21. Linnarsson, D.: Dynamics of pulmonary gas exchange and heart rate at start and end of exercise. Acta Physiol. Scand. **415**(suppl), 1–68 (1974)
22. Poole, D.C., Jones, A.M.: Oxygen uptake kinetics. Compr. Physiol. **2**, 933–996 (2012)
23. Rossiter, H.B.: Exercise: kinetic considerations for gas exchange. Compr. Physiol. **1**, 203–244 (2011)
24. Swanson, G.D.: Breath-to-breath considerations for gas exchange kinetics. In: Cerretelli, P., Whipp, B. (eds.) Exercise bioenergetics and gas exchange, pp. 211–222. Elsevier/North Holland, Amsterdam (1980)
25. Vogiatzis, I., et al.: Oxygen kinetics and debt during recovery from expiratory flow-limited exercise in healthy humans. Eur. J. Appl. Physiol. **99**, 265–274 (2007)
26. Wessel, H.U., Stout, R.L., Bastanier, C.K., Paul, M.H.: Breath-by-breath variation of FRC: effect on $\dot{V}O2$ and $\dot{V}CO2$ measured at the mouth. J. Appl. Physiol. **46**, 1122–1126 (1979)
27. West, J.B.: Regional differences in gas exchange in the lung of erect man. J. Appl. Physiol. **17**, 893–898 (1962)
28. Whipp, B.J., Ward, S.A., Rossiter, H.B.: Pulmonary O_2 uptake during exercise: conflating muscular and cardiovascular responses. Med. Sci. Sports Exerc. **37**, 1574–1585 (2005)
29. Wüst, R.C.I., Aliverti, A., Capelli, C., Kayser, B.: Breath-by-breath changes of lung oxygen stores at rest and during exercise in humans. Resp. Physiol. Neurobiol. **164**, 291–299 (2008)

The Application of Multiview Human Body Tracking on the Example of Hurdle Clearance

Tomasz Krzeszowski[1]([⊠]), Krzysztof Przednowek[2], Krzysztof Wiktorowicz[1], and Janusz Iskra[3]

[1] Faculty of Electrical and Computer Engineering,
Rzeszów University of Technology, Wincentego Pola 2, 35-959 Rzeszów, Poland
{tkrzeszo,kwiktor}@prz.edu.pl
[2] Faculty of Physical Education, University of Rzeszów,
Towarnickiego 3, 35-959 Rzeszów, Poland
krzprz@ur.edu.pl
[3] Faculty of Physical Education and Physiotherapy, Opole University of Technology,
Prószkowska 76, 45-758 Opole, Poland
j.iskra@awf.katowice.pl

Abstract. This initial research presents the multiview human body tracking method as a tool to measure hurdle clearance parameters. This study was conducted on high level hurdlers, who were members of the Polish national team. The video sequences were recorded by a multicamera system consisting of three 100 Hz Full HD cameras. The sequences were registered under the simulated starting conditions of a 110 m hurdles race. Kinematic parameters were estimated based on the analysis of images from the multicamera system. These parameters were compared with the parameters obtained from ground truth poses. Mean absolute error and mean relative error were selected as the quality criteria. The main advantage of the method presented here is that it does not need any special clothes, markers or the support of other estimation techniques.

Keywords: 110 m hurdles race · Human motion tracking ·
Multicamera system · Particle swarm optimization

1 Introduction

Hurdling is a group of athletic competitions in which technical preparation is very important. The hurdle race refers to running over 10 hurdles that are from 0.84 to 1.07 m high, depending on the event. Evaluation of hurdling technique is mainly focused on certain phases of human motion [1]. For example, the studies [2,3] are devoted to the kinematic analysis of the so called "hurdle clearance". The paper by Čoh [2] analyzes selected kinematic parameters (e.g., the height of center of mass, the leg angle) that describe the Colin Jackson's hurdle clearance technique. Salo et al. [4] present a three-dimensional (3D) biomechanical

© Springer Nature Switzerland AG 2019
J. Cabri et al. (Eds.): icSPORTS 2016/2017, CCIS 975, pp. 116–127, 2019.
https://doi.org/10.1007/978-3-030-14526-2_8

analysis of sprint hurdles. To estimate the parameters (e.g., the take-off distance, the horizontal velocity), two cameras with "Kine analysis" software were used. The main objective of this paper was to determine and compare selected biomechanical parameters of male and female athletes at different competitive levels.

One of the methods in supporting sports training is computer vision that plays an increasingly important role. For example, Reyes et al. [5] developed an algorithm that processes underwater video sequences for swimmer detection and tracking. The algorithm was tested on two video sequences. Motion detection and tracking methods are also described in the papers [6,7] where they were used to analyze athletics videos. Other solutions that use computer vision techniques are the systems for tracking players in indoor team games, such as handball [8] and basketball [9]. In the paper by Kwon et al. [9], a new multiple target tracking method based on the kernelised correlation filter was proposed. Indoor sports have also been analyzed by Kim and Cho [10], where the authors propose a robust multi-object tracking algorithm for acquiring object oriented multi-angle videos. In their algorithm, multiple camera images are integrated using homography-based transformation in order to cover large areas of interest. The papers [11,12] introduce algorithms for players' tracking in broadcast soccer videos. In [11], Manafifard et al. present an implementation of the appearance-based multiple hypothesis tracking algorithm. The authors utilized a particle swarm optimization to account for appearances, nonlinear movements and occlusions. Yang and Li [12] used a salient region detection to segment sports fields and edge detection combined with Otsu algorithm to detect soccer players. They used an enhanced particle filter for players' tracking. Markerless motion cupture systems for tracking of tennis racket is presented in [13] and [14]. For example, Sheets et al. [14] present a system to evaluate kinematic differences between the flat, kick, and slice serves. In this study, seven male players were tested on an outdoor court in daylight conditions. A method to identify sports players in videos has been proposed in [15], where the identification was achieved by motion feature matching between (unknown) players in videos (the features were obtained from estimated postures in the videos) and wearable sensors. The results of the experiment showed that the proposed method successfully identified 10 players with 72% accuracy. Cheng et al. [16] shown that the proposed motion descriptor could successfully classify the following four sports types: sprint, long-distance running, hurdling and canoeing. The results of the experiment were obtained by using video material from the 1992 Barcelona Olympic Games. The paper by Zhang et al. [17] proposes an algorithm to track athlete's actions from a sports video sequence. The presented method combines a particle filtering and mean shift in order to effectively trace a fast-moving target.

In this paper, a multiview markerless method of human body motion tracking is proposed. The developed system is used to estimate hurdle clearance parameters. In our analysis, eight angle parameters and nine distance parameters are taken into account. These parameters are estimated using image sequences captured by a multicamera system. In the tracking process, our method uses a particle swarm optimization algorithm. This study is an extended version of the former paper [18].

2   Methods

2.1   Multiview Human Motion Tracking

The purpose of human body tracking is to estimate a model that is close to real body pose as much as possible. The body pose is defined as the position and orientation of the model in space as well as the angles between the joints. It should be emphasized that capturing the 3D pose of a human body is a very difficult task [19, 20]. The main problems include: variability in the appearance of the tracked humans and environment, complexity of human motion, obscuring parts of the body, high dimensional search space and image noise. Although there are many different propositions to solve these problems, the most common use simplified human body models [19–22] or uniform background [21]. In the process of tracking, a particle filter algorithm [23] or its modified versions are frequently used [21]. However, these algorithms require a significant number of particles in order to find the correct solution, which affects the execution time. Therefore, in the human body motion tracking process, particle swarm optimization algorithms [19, 20, 22, 24] are used because they provide a more effective exploration of the search space.

In human body tracking, a 3D model is applied to determine the human body pose. The model used in this research is based on a kinematic tree structure consisting of 11 segments [18], each of which is represented by a truncated cone [20, 21]. The size of the space is determined by the number of degrees of freedom (DoF). Each segment includes up to three DoFs that define its orientation; the only exception is the pelvis, which contains three additional segments defining the model translation. The model used in this paper includes 24 DoFs. In our method, both the model and the body pose in the first frame of a image sequence are selected manually.

A particle swarm optimization algorithm (PSO) [22, 24] is used in the motion tracking process. In our proposition, a swarm particle represents the hypothetical state (pose) of an athlete. Each ith particle is described by its current position $\mathbf{x}_i$, velocity $\mathbf{v}_i$, and its best position $\mathbf{pbest}_i$. Moreover, all particles have access to the best global position $\mathbf{gbest}$, which has been found by any particle in the swarm. The velocity and the position of each particle are updated using the following equations:

$$\mathbf{v}_i^{k+1} = \chi[\mathbf{v}_i^k + c_1\mathbf{r}_1(\mathbf{pbest}_i - \mathbf{x}_i^k) + c_2\mathbf{r}_2(\mathbf{gbest} - \mathbf{x}_i^k)], \tag{1}$$

$$\mathbf{x}_i^{k+1} = \mathbf{x}_i^k + \mathbf{v}_i^{k+1}, \tag{2}$$

where $\chi = 0.75$ is the constriction factor, $\mathbf{r}_1$, $\mathbf{r}_2$ are uniformly distributed random numbers in the interval $[0, 1]$, and $c_1 = c_2 = 2.05$. The best solution is selected on the basis of a fitness function, that determines the degree of similarity between the estimated and the real human pose. The fitness function consists of two components. The first component is determined by using the extracted human silhouette, whereas the second is based on the edge distance map [19,22]. The value of the function for the cth camera is calculated using the following equation [18]:

$$f^c(\mathbf{x}) = 1 - (af_1^c(\mathbf{x}) + bf_2^c(\mathbf{x})) \tag{3}$$

where $\mathbf{x}$ is the human body pose (the position of a particle) and a, b are experimentally chosen factors. The function $f_1^c(\mathbf{x})$ describes the degree of overlap of the rendered 3D model with the extracted silhouette, and $f_2^c(\mathbf{x})$ is determined by comparing the 3D model edges with the image, including the map with pixel distances from the nearest edge. The fitness function for all cameras is determined according to the following equation [18]:

$$f(\mathbf{x}) = \frac{1}{C} \sum_{c=1}^{C} f^c(\mathbf{x}) \tag{4}$$

where $C = 3$ is the number of cameras.

2.2 Data Acquisition

The proposed method was applied for four image sequences obtained by recording two runs of two athletes. The athletes were the members of the Polish national team. The data were recorded in the athletics hall with a tartan track. In the research, the sequences of clearing the third hurdle in the regulation conditions of 110 m race (hurdle height: 1.067 m, distance between the hurdles: 9.14 m) were captured. The sequences, in the form of color images of size 1920×1080, were captured with the frequency of 100 Hz by three Basler Ace acA1920-150uc cameras. Figure 1 illustrates how the cameras were arranged in the athletics hall. The parameters of the cameras were estimated using the TSAI calibration method [25].

2.3 Evaluation of the Parameters

In our research, five key points (P_1–P_5) were analysed in three phases of hurdle clearance. The analysis included 17 parameters presented in Fig. 2. These parameters were selected based on the literature review [1,2]. The quality of tracking was evaluated using the estimated pose and the ground truth pose. The ground truth pose was obtained by manually matching the 3D model to the images of athletes that contained the five key poses characteristic for hurdle clearance (Fig. 2).

For each parameter the error level was determined. The parameters were estimated by the proposed algorithm and compared with the values of the ground truth reference model. The quality criterion for the nth repetition of the algorithm was defined as:

$$e_n = |\hat{X}_n - X| \tag{5}$$

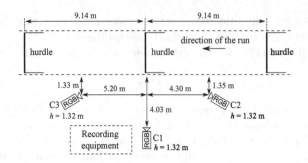

Fig. 1. Acquisition station, h is the height of the camera from the ground [18].

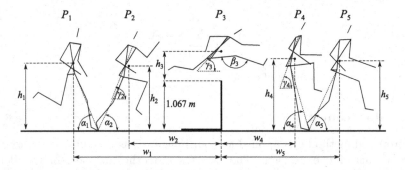

Fig. 2. Key points and parameters of hurdle clearance: P_1 is the braking point in take-off phase, P_2 is the propulsion point in take-off phase, P_3 is the center of mass (CM) over the hurdle in flight phase, P_4 is the braking point in landing phase, P_5 is the propulsion point in landing phase, h_1 is the height of CM, w_1 is the CM to hurdle distance, α_1 is the angle of the trail leg, h_2 is the height of CM, w_2 is the CM to hurdle distance, α_2 is the angle of the trail leg, γ_2 is the angle of inclination of the torso, h_3 is the height of CM (over the hurdle), β_3 is the angle of bend in the lead leg, γ_3 is the angle of inclination of the torso, h_4 is the height of CM, w_4 is the CM to hurdle distance, α_4 is the angle of the lead leg, γ_4 is the angle of inclination of the torso, h_5 is the height of CM, w_5 is the CM to hurdle distance, and α_5 is the angle of the lead leg [18].

$$\Delta = \frac{1}{N} \sum_{n=1}^{N} e_n \tag{6}$$

where e_n is the absolute error, $\hat{X}_n$ is the estimated value (determined by the algorithm), X is the ground truth value, Δ is the mean absolute error, and N is the number of algorithm repetitions. Moreover, the mean relative error was calculated from the following formula:

$$\delta = \frac{1}{N} \sum_{n=1}^{N} \frac{e_n}{X} \cdot 100 \tag{7}$$

3 Results of the Experiment

The multiview human motion tracking method was applied to four image sequences of two hurdles runners. The results were obtained by the PSO algorithm using 500 particles and 20 iterations. The examples of the tracking results for sequence 1 and sequence 3 for three views are shown in Figs. 3 and 4, respectively. The projected 3D model matches the athletes in the images reasonably well. However, some differences in relation to the ground truth poses can be observed (see, for example, Fig. 3, frame #39, 57, 65, and Fig. 4, frame #38, 57, 65). It should be mentioned that the algorithm sometimes 'loses' one or more parts of the body (tracking has failed), but it is usually able to correct this error in subsequent frames and estimate the correct posture. The problems mentioned are mainly due to occlusions, high dimensional search space and the errors in cameras calibration process.

The mean value for the analyzed parameters and the ground truth value X are presented in Table 1. The parameters were obtained for 10 repetitions of the tracking algorithm. The calculated parameters describe the technique of clearing the hurdle in five key points (P_1–P_5). For example, for hurdler 1 in sequence 1, it is noted that the height of the center of mass at individual points of a hurdling step is respectively $h_1 = 959\,\text{mm}$, $h_2 = 1065\,\text{mm}$, $h_4 = 1103\,\text{mm}$ and $h_5 = 1042\,\text{mm}$. At point P_3, when the hurdler is over the hurdle, the height of the CM is highest and in respect to the hurdle is $h_3 = 241.1\,\text{mm}$. Another parameter characterizing the technique is the inclination angle of the torso γ. This parameter at P_2 has the highest value ($72.4°$) and the lowest at P_4 ($53.9°$). A characteristic angle when analyzing the hurdle step is the angle of bend in the lead leg in the flight phase (β). This angle for hurdler 1 in sequence 1 is $137.7°$. The parameters w_1, w_2, w_4 and w_5 describe the center of mass distance from the hurdle. For example, the value of w_1 for competitor 1 in sequence 1 indicates that P_1 lies approx. 2567 mm before the hurdle.

Table 2 presents the errors Δ and δ. The error analysis shows that among all the distance parameters, the estimation of CM height over hurdle in P_3 (h_3) for all sequences is determined with the greatest δ error. This error is the largest for sequence 1 ($\delta = 19.1\%$ and $\Delta = 56.7\,\text{mm}$). In the case of sequence 3, this error is the smallest and equal to 11.2% ($\Delta = 32.7$ mm). Krzeszowski et al. [22] used a monocular motion tracking system, and this parameter was determined with $\bar{\Delta} = 30.5\,\text{mm}$ and $\bar{\delta} = 8.3\%$. The smallest δ error for all sequences is obtained for the CM distance from the hurdle in P_1 (w_1). This error is equal to 1.0% ($\Delta = 25.7\,\text{mm}$) in sequence 2 and it is equal to 0.4% ($\Delta = 10.0\,\text{mm}$) in sequence 3. In the work [22], the errors for w_1 were $\bar{\Delta} = 25.8$ mm and $\bar{\delta} = 1.0\%$. By analyzing the angular errors it can be seen that the smallest mean error for all sequences $\bar{\delta}$ was obtained for the angle of the trail leg in P_2 (α_2) and it is equal to 2.1% ($\bar{\Delta} = 2.4°$). The error δ is the smallest in sequence 3 ($\delta = 1.3\%$ and $\Delta = 1.4°$). The angle of inclination of the torso in P_3 (γ_3) is determined

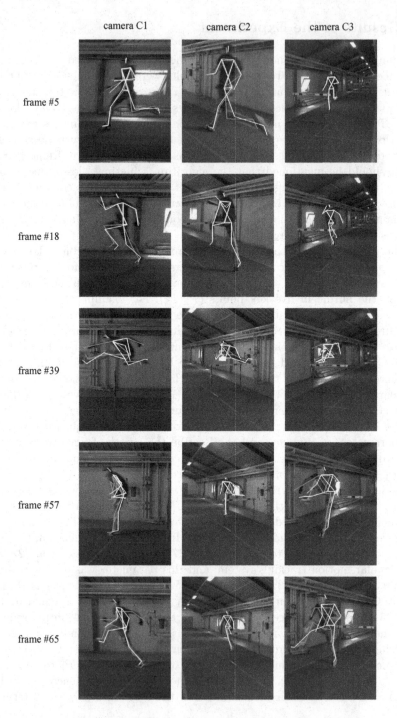

Fig. 3. Example of tracking results on sequence 1; the green skeleton is the ground truth pose and the white skeleton is the estimated pose. (Color figure online)

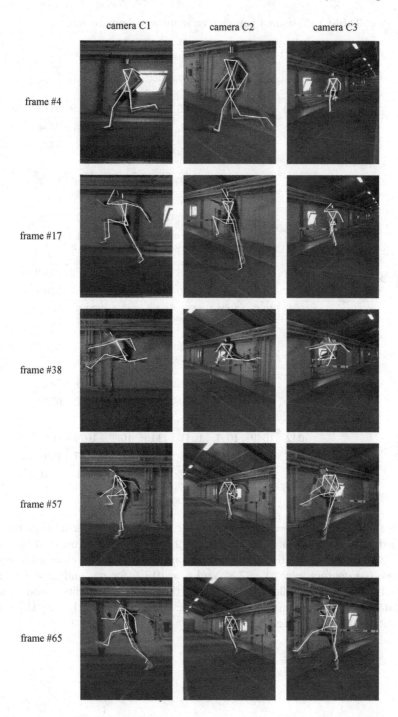

Fig. 4. Example of tracking results on sequence 3; the green skeleton is the ground truth pose and the white skeleton is the estimated pose. (Color figure online)

Table 1. Measured parameters; units: h, w [mm], α, γ, β [°].

Parameter	Seq. 1		Seq. 2		Seq. 3		Seq. 4	
	$\bar{x}$	X	$\bar{x}$	X	$\bar{x}$	X	$\bar{x}$	X
P_1								
h_1	959.0	959.1	952.7	953.5	929.3	933.2	949.9	937.3
w_1	2567	2549	2528	2502	2677	2667	2735	2734
α_1	64.9	61.4	66.8	62.4	64.3	62.9	66.8	64.9
P_2								
h_2	1065	1130	1123	1159	1083	1139	1094	1147
w_2	1689	1605	1569	1525	1748	1677	1875	1760
α_2	71.2	72.0	69.6	67.2	67.9	69.0	68.0	70.9
γ_2	72.4	75.9	75.6	74.9	74.6	75.9	75.4	75.9
P_3								
h_3	241.1	297.9	235.1	280.8	265.6	292.4	269.2	295.2
β_3	137.7	164.0	141.1	164.0	150.1	164.0	152.1	170.1
γ_3	59.8	40.8	59.9	40.8	64.2	48.1	72.5	50.1
P_4								
h_4	1103	1100	1066	1098	1142	1159	1115	1115
w_4	1224	1296	1105	1175	1253	1234	1135	1125
α_4	70.2	68.0	70.8	70.4	69.0	73.0	73.5	75.0
γ_4	53.9	65.8	51.8	65.8	52.4	67.6	63.7	67.6
P_5								
h_5	1042	1049	1057	1041	1118	1089	1074	1067
w_5	1823	1809	1676	1683	1825	1813	1577	1594
α_5	74.9	70.0	84.7	70.0	77.2	65.0	74.4	71.0

with the greatest error $\bar{\delta} = 43.0\%$ ($\bar{\Delta} = 19.2°$). This parameter in sequence 1 is obtained with the error $\delta = 46.7\%$ ($\Delta = 19.1°$), while in sequence 3 the error is $\delta = 33.5\%$ and $\Delta = 16.1°$. In the previous work [22], the estimation errors for these parameters were $\bar{\Delta} = 7.8°$ and $\bar{\delta} = 10.1\%$ for α_2, and $\bar{\Delta} = 5.9°$ and $\bar{\delta} = 12.1\%$ for γ_3. It should be emphasised that the mean errors $\bar{\delta}$ and $\bar{\Delta}$ were calculated for four sequences in this paper, while in the work [22], the errors were obtained for 10 sequences.

Table 2. Errors; units: h, w [mm], α, γ, β [°], $\delta, \bar{\delta}$ [%].

Parameter	Seq. 1		Seq. 2		Seq. 3		Seq. 4		Mean	
	Δ	δ	Δ	δ	Δ	δ	Δ	δ	$\bar{\Delta}$	$\bar{\delta}$
P_1										
h_1	8.4	0.9	10.0	1.1	14.8	1.6	13.1	1.4	11.6	1.3
w_1	17.6	0.7	25.7	1.0	10.0	0.4	20.3	0.7	18.4	0.7
α_1	3.5	5.6	4.5	7.2	2.3	3.7	3.0	4.6	3.3	5.3
P_2										
h_2	64.7	5.7	36.3	3.1	56.3	4.9	55.5	4.8	53.2	4.6
w_2	83.6	5.2	44.0	2.9	71.3	4.3	115.0	6.5	78.5	4.7
α_2	1.7	1.6	3.4	3.0	1.4	1.3	2.9	2.7	2.4	2.1
γ_2	3.5	4.7	1.5	2.0	3.3	4.4	1.7	2.2	2.5	3.3
P_3										
h_3	56.7	19.1	48.2	17.2	32.7	11.2	38.2	12.9	44.0	15.1
β_3	26.3	16.0	23.0	14.0	15.3	9.3	17.9	10.5	20.6	12.5
γ_3	19.1	46.7	19.1	46.8	16.1	33.5	22.5	44.8	19.2	43.0
P_4										
h_4	21.1	1.9	38.4	3.5	59.7	5.1	31.3	2.8	37.6	3.3
w_4	72.3	5.6	69.2	5.9	36.5	2.9	28.1	2.4	51.5	4.2
α_4	3.9	5.7	4.6	6.5	5.8	8.0	1.7	2.2	4.0	5.6
γ_4	11.8	17.9	13.9	21.1	15.4	22.8	4.8	7.1	11.5	17.2
P_5										
h_5	30.6	2.9	56.0	5.4	54.3	5.0	48.1	4.0	47.3	4.3
w_5	48.9	2.7	49.0	2.9	65.3	3.6	28.2	1.0	47.9	2.6
α_5	5.2	7.4	14.7	21.0	12.3	18.9	5.4	7.6	9.4	13.7

4 Conclusions

This paper proposed a multiview markerless method to track human body motion. The experiments were performed on four image sequences of two athletes clearing a hurdle. The estimated parameters were compared with the parameters calculated from ground truth poses that were obtained in the manual manner. The conducted error analysis indicates that the results are promising, but further research is necessary. At the current stage of the research, the proposed method has some limitations. These limitations are related to the accuracy of the pose estimation and the complicated calibration procedure of the multi-camera system.

Our future work will focus on improvement of the proposed method and its modification for computing on mobile devices. We will also concentrate on using this method in practice to support technical preparation of athletes.

Acknowledgements. This work has been partially supported by the Polish Ministry of Science and Higher Education within the research project "Development of Academic Sport" in the years 2016-2018, project No. N RSA4 00554.

References

1. Iskra, J.: Scientific research in hurdle races. AWF Katowice (2012)
2. Čoh, M.: Biomechanical analysis of Colin Jackson's hurdle clearance technique. New Studi. Athletics **1**, 33–40 (2003)
3. Čoh, M., Dolenec, A., Tomažin, K., Zvan, M.: Dynamic and kinematic analysis of the hurdle clearance technique. In: Čoh, M. (ed.) Biomechanical Diagnostic Methods in Athletic Training. University of Ljubljana, pp. 109–116 (2008)
4. Salo, A., Grimshaw, P.N., Marar, L.: 3-D biomechanical analysis of sprint hurdles at different competitive levels. Med. Sci. Sports Exerc. **29**, 231–237 (1997)
5. Reyes, C.E., Mojica, E.F., Correa, C.V., Arguello, H.: Algorithm for underwater swimmer tracking using the HSV color model and compressive sensing. In: 2016 IEEE Colombian Conference on Communications and Computing (COLCOM), pp. 1–5 (2016)
6. Ramasso, E., Panagiotakis, C., Rombaut, M., Pellerin, D., Tziritas, G.: Human shape-motion analysis in athletics videos for coarse to fine action/activity recognition using transferable belief model. Electron. Lett. Comput. Vis. Image Anal. **7**, 32–50 (2009)
7. Panagiotakis, C., Grinias, I., Tziritas, G.: Automatic human motion analysis and action recognition in athletics videos. In: 14th European Signal Processing Conference, pp. 1–5 (2006)
8. Perš, J., Kovacic, S.: A system for tracking players in sports games by computer vision. Elektrotehniški vestnik **67**, 281–288 (2000)
9. Kwon, J., Kim, K., Cho, K.: Multi-target tracking by enhancing the kernelised correlation filter-based tracker. Electron. Lett. **53**, 1358–1360 (2017)
10. Kim, Y., Cho, K.S.: Robust multi-object tracking to acquire object oriented videos in indoor sports. In: 2016 International Conference on Information and Communication Technology Convergence (ICTC), pp. 1104–1107 (2016)
11. Manafifard, M., Ebadi, H., Moghaddam, H.A.: Appearance-based multiple hypothesis tracking: application to soccer broadcast videos analysis. Sig. Process.: Image Commun. **55**, 157–170 (2017)
12. Yang, Y., Li, D.: Robust player detection and tracking in broadcast soccer video based on enhanced particle filter. J. Vis. Commun. Image Represent. **46**, 81–94 (2017)
13. Elliott, N., Choppin, S., Goodwill, S.R., Allen, T.: Markerless tracking of tennis racket motion using a camera. Procedia Eng. **72**, 344–349 (2014). The Engineering of Sport 10
14. Sheets, A.L., Abrams, G.D., Corazza, S., Safran, M.R., Andriacchi, T.P.: Kinematics differences between the flat, kick, and slice serves measured using a markerless motion capture method. Ann. Biomed. Eng. **39**, 3011–3020 (2011)
15. Hamatani, T., Sakaguchi, Y., Uchiyama, A., Higashino, T.: Player identification by motion features in sport videos using wearable sensors. In: 2016 Ninth International Conference on Mobile Computing and Ubiquitous Networking (ICMU), pp. 1–6 (2016)

16. Cheng, F., Christmas, W., Kittler, J.: Periodic human motion description for sports video databases. In: Proceedings of the Pattern Recognition, 17th International Conference on ICPR 2004, vol. 3, pp. 870–873. IEEE Computer Society, Washington, DC (2004)

17. Zhang, Y., Feng, S., Sun, X., Yang, H.: Research on tracking algorithm for fast-moving target in sport video. J. Comput. Theor. Nanosci. **14**, 230–236 (2017)

18. Krzeszowski, T., Przednowek, K., Wiktorowicz, K., Iskra, J.: Multiview human body tracking of hurdle clearance: a case study. In: Proceedings of the 5th International Congress on Sport Sciences Research and Technology Support, vol. 1, pp. 83–88. icSPORTS, INSTICC, SciTePress (2017)

19. John, V., Trucco, E., Ivekovic, S.: Markerless human articulated tracking using hierarchical particle swarm optimisation. Image Vis. Comput. **28**, 1530–1547 (2010)

20. Kwolek, B., Krzeszowski, T., Gagalowicz, A., Wojciechowski, K., Josinski, H.: Real-time multi-view human motion tracking using particle swarm optimization with resampling. In: Perales, F.J., Fisher, R.B., Moeslund, T.B. (eds.) AMDO 2012. LNCS, vol. 7378, pp. 92–101. Springer, Heidelberg (2012). https://doi.org/10.1007/978-3-642-31567-1_9

21. Deutscher, J., Reid, I.: Articulated body motion capture by stochastic search. Int. J. Comput. Vision **61**, 185–205 (2005)

22. Krzeszowski, T., Przednowek, K., Wiktorowicz, K., Iskra, J.: Estimation of hurdle clearance parameters using a monocular human motion tracking method. Comput. Methods Biomech. Biomed. Eng. **19**, 1319–1329 (2016). PMID: 26838547

23. Sidenbladh, H., Black, M.J., Fleet, D.J.: Stochastic tracking of 3D human figures using 2D image motion. In: Vernon, D. (ed.) ECCV 2000. LNCS, vol. 1843, pp. 702–718. Springer, Heidelberg (2000). https://doi.org/10.1007/3-540-45053-X_45

24. Kennedy, J., Eberhart, R.: Particle swarm optimization. In: Proceedings of IEEE International Conference on Neural Networks, vol. 4, pp. 1942–1948. IEEE Press, Piscataway (1995)

25. Tsai, R.: A versatile camera calibration technique for high-accuracy 3D machine vision metrology using off-the-shelf TV cameras and lenses. IEEE J. Robot. Autom. **3**, 323–344 (1987)

Study on Game Information Analysis
for Support to Tactics and Strategies
in Curling

Fumito Masui[1(✉)], Hiromu Otani[2], Hitoshi Yanagi[1,3], and Michal Ptaszynski[4]

[1] Research Centre for Winter Sports Science, Kitami Institute of Technology,
165, Kouen-cho, Kitami, Japan
ice@ialab.cs.kitami-it.ac.jp
[2] KYOCERA Communication Systems Co., Ltd.,
6, Takeda Tobadono-cho, Fushimi-ku, Kyoto, Japan
[3] High Performance Committee, Japan Curling Association,
1-1-1, Jin-nan, Shibuya-ku, Tokyo, Japan
[4] School of Regional Innovation and Social Design Engineering,
Kitami Institute of Technology, 165, Kouen-cho, Kitami, Japan

Abstract. Curling is a winter sport often referred to as "chess on ice". There are three factors influencing game performance in this game: physical factor, human factor, and strategic/tactical factor. The strategic/tactical factor is considered as the most important at the top level. In this paper, we report on new knowledge we obtained regarding the relationship between shot accuracy and difference in game score, and difference in correlation for each level in 378 games, covering around 60,000 shots as a research subject of Curling Informatics project.

Keywords: Curling Informatics · Digital scorebook ·
Tactics and strategies · Game information · Game score ·
Shot accuracy · Sochi Winter Olympics

1 Introduction

It is still fresh news for Japanese winter sports fans that Japan national curling team won second place at the Women's World Championship 2016 in Saskatchewan, Canada, thus winning a medal for the first time. Curling is a winter sport confirmed to be in existence from several hundred years ago[1]. Japan women team has participated in Olympic curling since it became an official Olympic sport in 1998. Moreover, in the Pyeongchang Winter Olympics in 2018, both the men's and women's teams qualified to play for the first time in 20 years.

Due to rise in both the level of play of curling players and the popularity of curling game in Japan it is still necessary to continue working on strengthening the support in order to make Japan capable of obtaining a medal at

---

[1] For example, the painting in the Snow by Pieter Bruegel in 1565 depicts people enjoying playing curling on a frozen lake.

© Springer Nature Switzerland AG 2019
J. Cabri et al. (Eds.): icSPORTS 2016/2017, CCIS 975, pp. 128–149, 2019.
https://doi.org/10.1007/978-3-030-14526-2_9

the Pyeongchang Winter Olympics in 2018. For example, Japan played against Switzerland three times till now, including round robin (type of tournament in which every team competes against every other team in turns). This suggests that Japan should have already captured the tactics of the Swiss team which should help in winning a gold medal or at least improve the team's ranking during the Pyeongchang Winter Olympics.

Factors influencing team's performance in curling include: the physical factor (ice condition), the human factor (condition of curling player), and the strategic/tactical factor (knowledge of tactics/strategies). Bradley [1] points out the strategic/tactical factor as the most important at the top level.

There are various strengthening programs developed for strengthening of Japanese curling [2–4]. An information science approach can be mentioned as an example of a method for improving the performance of a team. In the past few years a number of cases to support sports with ICT (Information and Communication Technology) have been reported [5,6], including curling [4].

As strengthening programs regarding the strategic/tactical factor, our group proposed a new field called *Curling Informatics* [4]. As Fig. 1 shows, the research field of Curling Informatics deals with strategic and tactical factors of curling teams and improves the strategic and tactical skills of curling players.

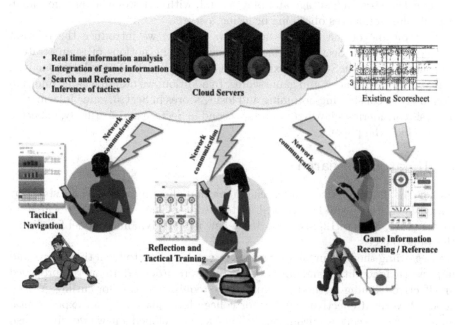

Fig. 1. The concept of Curling Informatics [4].

Specifically, general plan developed within this field aims at implementing the methods to (1) collect, (2) analyze, (3) visualize and (4) share game information.

In the first step, Masui et al. developed a digital scorebook iCE which runs on a tablet computer to collect and analyze game information and they confirmed validity of the system [7,8]. This system realized (1), (3) and part of (2), and aims to realize point (4) right now. In addition, it is come up to practical use and 11 teams of Japanese national top level have been using this application.

iCE allows checking shot accuracy of each team or player based on collected information sequentially and visually.

Additionally, iCE compiles a shot score database from basic data of shot accuracy, which makes it possible to organize and analyze scores from a variety of viewpoints [4,8,9]. To grasp the characteristics and trends for each teams we analyzed the information on shot scores in more detail. And this in result lead us to finding a difference in strategy between a rival country and Japan in an objective way.

As a part of Curling Informatics project, in this study we manually analyzed game information with the aim to specify the team's characteristics and establish the appropriate analytical method.

In this paper, we discuss the influence of shot accuracy on game result by focusing on the relationship between shot accuracy and game score. Specifically, we perform three research tasks: verification of the usefulness of the previous method, analysis of influence of the starting position (later called: play first, without last stone advantage and play second, with last stone advantage), analysis of what influences obtaining or losing a score.

The outline of the paper is as follows. Firstly, we introduce the relevant related research in Sect. 2. Secondly, we describe the notions of team strategy and shot accuracy in Sect. 3. Next, we provide an overview of correlation analysis between shot accuracies and game scores. In addition, we describe game information analysis considering obtaining and losing scores in Sect. 5, game information analysis considering play first and play second in Sects. 6 and 7. Finally, in Sect. 8 we conclude the paper.

2   Related Research

As for the human factor, research on motion dynamics of curling stone by Shegelski et al. [10] and Denny et al. [11] are some of the most known research. In recent years, Maeno [12] also reported a new motion dynamics model for sliding the stone on ice.

Regarding the human factor, various research on how to train the players and improve their condition and power balancing, were proposed. Behm [13] proposed an effective training method to improve the requisite motion for curling. Yanagi et al. [2] verified effective training for college level players by an experimental approach with a college curling team. They also developed a new sweeping brush which conveys the power of player's motion effectively based on the analysis of player's sweeping motions from a viewpoint of biomechanics.

In addition, Tanaka [14] introduced ICT for human factor analysis. They attempted to carry out an analysis of motion to deliver the stone by utilizing a virtual model of curling environment and players.

About the strategic/tactical factor, Igarashi et al. [15] proposed an application to inverse the problem for curling by policy-gradient methods in Non-Markov decision processes, Ura et al. [16] reported on calculation technique for analysis of strategies/tactics based on the game tree. Also, Sung et al. [17] analyzed game information focusing on first stone and last stone per each end and points out that team strategies/tactics differed in teams which had last stone per end and other teams.

However, the goals of their results were not supportive enough for developing actual curling strategies and tactics, but rather they can be considered as works recognizing the problem and intensifying the need to find a solution. Moreover, they did not confirm the effectiveness of their methods in practice.

3   Team Strategies/Tactics and Shot Accuracy

Curling is a winter sport in which two teams compete to obtain points by throwing 16 stones at the center of a circular area called a *house* in an ice-based square area called a *sheet*. One team consists of four players. Each player throws two stones (called *shot*) in rotation, and the score is calculated by each rotation, till all 16 stones are thrown. At this time, the team that has a stone at the nearest position to the center of the house gets the number of points equal to the number of stones on the inside of the opponent's stones in the *house*. The scoring team was Play first in the next rotation. One rotation is called an *end*. One game consists of eight or ten ends, but the game is extended if the score is tied in the final end [18,19].

Curling is often called "chess on ice" because it is a sport in which tactics play an important role. It requires a player to form complex strategies in search for effective moves with consideration of ice condition, stone position in the *house*, etc.

Shots in curling are roughly divided into two types: *draw shot* and *takeout shot*. In *draw shots*, the stone stops in the *house*. *Takeout shots* force opponent stone out of the *house*. The thrown shot is given from 0 to 4 points by a team coach or a substitute player. In the special case, such as takeout shot that hits more opposite stone than advised by the skip, 5 points can be given. These points are called "*shot-score*", and shot accuracy (*SA*) is calculated using shot-score according to Eq. (1). SA has been one of the most important measurements to estimate player's skill and condition.

$$SA = 25 \times \frac{total\ of\ shot\text{-}scores}{number\ of\ shots}(\%) \tag{1}$$

The team which has a higher SA is in general capable to throw more accurate shots. Therefore, it gives an advantage to the team in the game. The team which has higher SA is more likely to succeed when performing the shot in critical situations. And the team which has lower SA would raise the probability for scoring by the opposite team.

This means that SA may be considered to scales that reflect skills of a team or player that carry out the strategies/tactics during the play. Therefore, by analyzing the relation between information of game score (GS) and SA, it could be possible to objectively examine the influence on game results by performance of team tactics.

Masui et al. [4] suggested that there is a strong correlation between the difference in SA and the difference in GS. In addition, they observed that Japanese national class is stronger than Japanese junior national class, and that the performance of Japanese national class is rarely influenced by missed shots. It means that the game result could be predicted before the game ends if we knew the difference in the playing teams' SA. Furthermore, the correlation in world class becomes weaker than the Japanese national class because of smaller differences in SA.

4 Correlation Analysis Between Shot Accuracy and Game Score

To verify the analysis of Masui et al. mentioned in Sect. 3, we analyzed the game information of world class teams in detail.

4.1 Analysis Procedure

Figure 2 shows the analysis procedure.

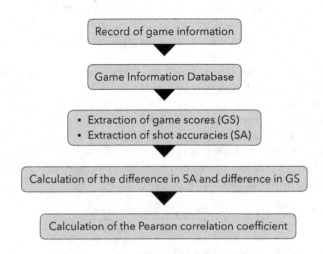

Fig. 2. Analysis procedure [20,21].

Firstly, we extracted the Difference in Final Game Scores ($DFGS$) and SA for each collected game from iCE's database.

Table 1. Target game information for analysis [20, 21].

Year	Championships	Number of games
2012	30th Japan Championship	26
	PACC Japan Palyoff	16
	Pacific Asia Junior Championship	20
	World Junior Championship	11
	3th College Championship	10
	Universiade 2013 of Japan Playoff	7
2013	Japan Junior Championship	24
	31th Japan Championship	11
	Olymipic Winter Games of Japan Playoff	21
	4th College Championship	11
2014	5th College Championship	13
	Universiade 2015 of Japan Playoff	30
	Advics Cup	13
	Sochi Olympic Winter Games	93
2015	World Woman's Championship	72
Total		378

Next, we calculated the difference in SA and Pearson's correlation coefficient based on extracted data. In addition, we examined a correlation between difference in GS and difference in SA.

By carrying out this analysis, it can be confirmed how much SA impacts game result. In addition, we compared the results separately for each player level, from which we expect extracting tendencies or tactical characteristics of each level.

4.2 Target Data

In this section, we describe target data used in analysis. As the target data we used the game information of 16 championships, 378 games covering around 60,000 shots[2]. Table 1 shows target game information for analysis in detail.

At recording game information, operator (2 or 3 persons) using 2 or 3 tablet-type devices with installed *iCE* application, 4 digital video cameras, 2 laptops in seats for recording data or photos. The movie taken by digital video camera was used for checking the recording data.

With regards to Sochi Olympic Winter Game (93 games), we extracted game information from *Curlit*[3] by the World Curling Federation and calculated SA unambiguously.

---

[2] It is larger than data used in Masui et al. (285 games covering around 45,000 shots).
[3] http://www.olympic.org/sochi-2014/curling.

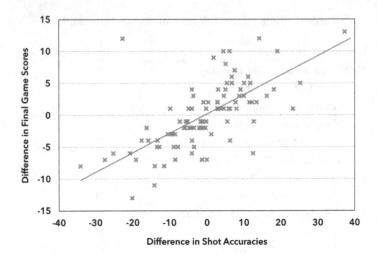

Fig. 3. Correlation between difference in shot accuracies vs. difference in final game scores for top level.

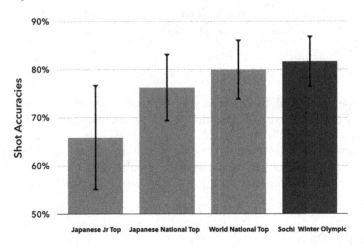

Fig. 4. Shot accuracy for each level.

4.3   Result and Discussion

In this section, we describe the relationship between differences in SA and DFGS for 387 games. The following presents the results for each player level.

Japanese Junior Top Level. Figure 3 shows a diagram representing a correlation between differences in SA, and DFGS and regression line for 126 games of Japanese junior top level. In Figure 3, the X axis shows difference in teams' shot accuracies each game and the Y axis represents the DFGS.

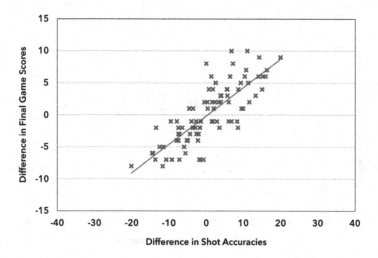

Fig. 5. Correlation between difference in shot accuracies vs. difference in final game scores for Japanese national top level.

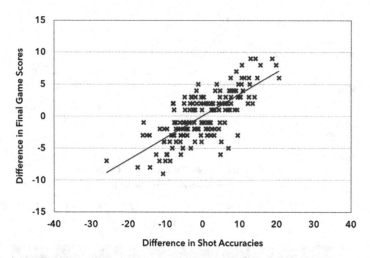

Fig. 6. Correlation between difference in shot accuracies vs. difference in final game scores for world national top level.

We calculated Pearson's correlation coefficient between difference in SA and DFGS, Japanese junior top level was 0.728.

In addition, we calculated team shot accuracies. Figure 4 shows team shot accuracies per player level. In Fig. 4, the X axis shows level, the Y axis shows SA for each game and the Error bar stands for standard deviation.

For Japanese junior top level, the results was $65.88\% \pm 10.95\,S.D.$

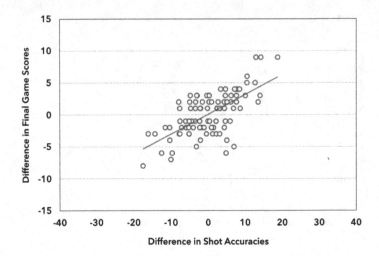

Fig. 7. Correlation between difference in shot accuracies vs. difference in final game scores for Sochi Winter Olympic Games.

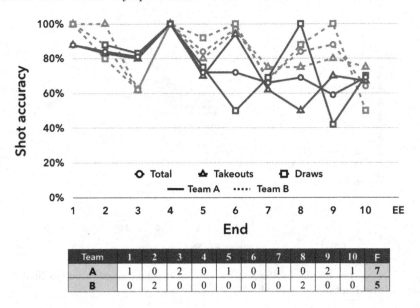

Team	1	2	3	4	5	6	7	8	9	10	F
A	1	0	2	0	1	0	1	0	2	1	7
B	0	2	0	0	0	0	0	2	0	0	5

Fig. 8. Team's shot accuracies for every ends and transition of game score (1) [20].

Japanese National Top Level. Figure 5 shows a diagram representing a correlation between difference in SA and DFGS and regression line for 87 games of Japanese national top level.

For Japanese national top level, the Pearson's correlation coefficient was 0.804 and team's SA was 76.21% ± 7.04 S.D. Both results were higher than Japanese junior top level.

World National Top Level. Figure 6 shows a diagram representing a correlation between difference in SA and DFGS and regression line for 165 games of World national top level.

The Pearson's correlation coefficient for two factors was 0.736. It is lower than Japanese national top level. On the other hand, team's SA was 80.28% ± 6.69 $S.D.$, higher level teams achieve higher SA and lower standard deviation.

Sochi Winter Olympic Games. Next, we describe the result of Sochi Winter Olympic Games. Figure 7 shows a diagram representing a correlation between difference in SA and DFGS and regression line for 93 newly collected games.

Pearson correlation coefficient between the two differences for total data was 0.667. This result was lower than the above mentioned Japanese junior top level, much less Japanese national top level. However, teams' SA was 82.01 ± 5.80$S.D.$ It was higher than Japanese national top level in Fig. 4. In other words, game information of world class teams indicated a very high SA. And yet the correlation between the two differences was low. These results were similar to those of Masui et al. This means that tactics or planning each end have an impact on a game result or difference in game score[4].

It could be possible that the correlation is negatively influenced by outliers. The more games containing outliers, the lower the correlation. It can be expected that we could expose the process of how tactics or strategies affect game result or difference in GS by analyzing the game of outliers.

Next, we analyzed two games in which the team of superior SA lost due to failure in tactics.

Figures 9 and 8 represent graphs showing transition of teams' SA for every end of each game. The X axis means the number of ends and the Y axis shows team's SA.

As shown in Fig. 9, game deployments do not indicate the difference in game scores until the middle of the game. While near the end of the game, team A gained multiple scores and won the game. As the rate of shots performed by each team, ratio of *takeout shots* for team A was 64% (51 shots in total of 80 shots) and ratio of *draw shots* was 36% (29 shots in total of 80 shots). Team A performed more takeouts than draws. On the other hand, ratio of *takeout shots* for team B was 51% (41 shots in total of 80 shots) and ratio of *draw shots* was 49% (39 shots in total of 80 shots). Team B performed similar number of *takeout* and *draw* shots. *Takeout shots* reduce the score probability of the opponent team because they force a stone out of the *house*. *Draw shots* raise the score probability of one's own team because they accumulate stone the *house*. In short, as the cause of victory it can be considered that team A took the tactics of risk aversion by performing selected *takeout shots* and accurately taking advantage of missed shots performed by team B. In fact, in the third end and ninth end, team A obtained their scores because the situation changed due to a missed shot of team B.

---

[4] For example, intentionally performing a missed shot.

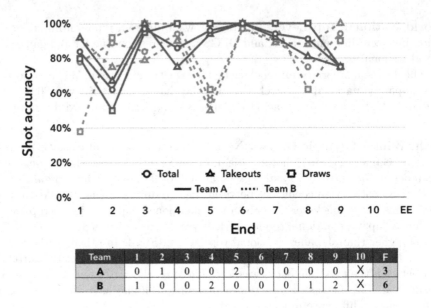

Team	1	2	3	4	5	6	7	8	9	10	F
A	0	1	0	0	2	0	0	0	0	X	3
B	1	0	0	2	0	0	0	1	2	X	6

Fig. 9. Team's shot accuracies for every ends and transition of game score (2) [20].

As Fig. 8 shows team A's draw SA is 100% from fourth end to eighth end. However, they made some scores only at the fifth end. Also in this game, team B which won the game had the *takeout shots* at 64% (49 shots in total of 76 shots) and the percentage of *draw shots* was 36% (27 shots in total of 76 shots). It means that team B performed more *takeouts* than *draws*. In game information of world class, the teams' shot accuracies exceed 80% and a standard deviation is small. It suggests that one missed shot can have an impact on the match situation more than in games of Japanese national top level. Also in this game, it can be considered that tactics of team B was based on purposeful exploiting missed shots of team A.

Therefore, as the cause of victory we can determine that team A took the tactics of risk aversion as their priority. Thus the selected tactics and a contributing shot and pressure for opponent had an impact on the game result.

However, this analysis did not consider the situations of obtaining or losing scores. The current analysis is using information GS and SA from 1 end to 10 end (in some cases, 11 end). It could contain confused information about tendencies in strategies or play characteristics among *Scoreless end* where both teams did not gain a score, *Get score end* that ended with gaining 1 or more, *Lose score end* that ended with obtaining a score by the opponent team.

Additionally, our analysis did not distinguish between the play first and play second. In general, the team that plays as the second has an advantage in curling because they can perform the last shot at an end. Accordingly, the strategies/tactics taken by each team differ depending on whether their playing position is played first or play second. In some cases, the strategies/tactics taken by the opposite team are advantageous. In other cases, it is necessary to take the opposite stone out of the house to set advantageous stone position, and put the stone in the house to get a higher score.

Therefore, to extract play characteristics in strategies in detail, it needs to perform analysis considering getting or losing scores and the order of teams in play.

5   Game Analysis Considering Get Score and Lose Score

To tackle the problem mentioned in Sect. 4, we added the parameter and analyzed game information again. This will be explained as game information analysis considering get score and lose score in this while game information analysis considering play first and play second will be explained in Sect. 6.

In this section, we formulated a hypothesis that "by considering get score and lose score, the correlation between SA and GS should rise", and verified the hypothesis in the following paragraphs of the paper based on the analysis of game information database.

5.1   Analysis Method and Target Data

This analysis adds a parameter of get score and lose score to the method described in Sect. 4.1.

Specifically, we exclude the end that target team did not gain any score (the score is zero) when we calculated the average of SA from 1 to 10 end. And then after that we calculated the average of SA again using end that target team gained a score or multiple scores. We defined Get Score Shot Accuracy (GS-SA) for this value. For example, in the game of Fig. 10, team A has gained at 2, 4, 7, 9 end. In this method, we extract the x2, x4, x7, x9 with SA of the above 4 ends, and calculate μ (the average value) of GS-SA.

A		1	2	3	4	5	6	7	8	9	10	Total Ave.
	GS	0	1	0	2	0	0	4	0	3	0	10
	SA(%)		X2		X4			X7		X9		μ

Fig. 10. Calculation examples of get score shot accuracy.

Next, we examined the correlation between DFGS and difference in GS-SA[5]. Additionally, we calculated Difference in Get Multiple Score Shot Accuracy ($DGMS$-SA) using ends that target team gained 2 or more by a similar technique, and examined the correlation between it and DFGS.

As the target data we used the game information of 93 games (45 games for men, 48 games for women) covering around 15,000 shots in Winter Olympic Games 2014 as game data of world national top level in Table 1.

---

[5] Hereinafter, this is called a Difference in Get Score Shot Accuracy (DGS-SA).

5.2   Result of Analysis

Here we describe the result of correlation between SA with get score and GS. Figure 11 shows a diagram representing a correlation between DGS-SA, and DFGS and regression line.

Pearson's correlation coefficient between the two differences for total data was 0.298, the two differences in Fig. 12 did not have any correlation. It means

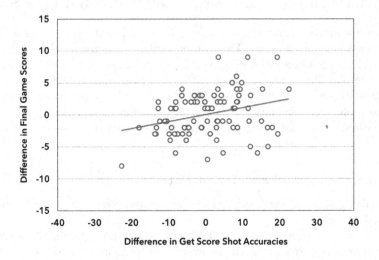

Fig. 11. Correlation between difference in get score shot accuracies vs. difference in final game scores.

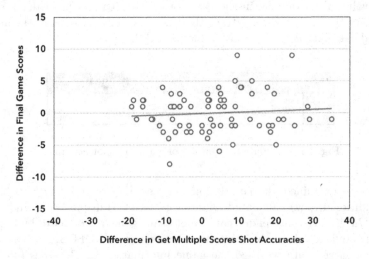

Fig. 12. Correlation between difference in get multiple scores shot accuracies vs. difference in final game scores.

that the SA didn't contribute to GS in getting score ends. Therefore, the success of shots did not involve GS.

Next, we describe the result of correlation between SA in getting multiple scores and GS. Further, we confirmed 19 games that target team did not gain multiple scores (the team gain zero or 1) in 10 ends. This information did not allow for calculation of GMS-SA. Because of that, we analyzed 74 games not including above 19 games as the target data.

Figure 12 shows a diagram representing a correlation between DGMS-SA, and DFGS and regression line.

The Pearson's correlation coefficient between the two differences for total data was 0.083. It is lower than the correlation for Sochi Winter Olympic Games mentioned in Sect. 4. Also, this result means that SA did not contribute to GS in the same manner as above.

From the above results, in world national top class, get score ends and lose score ends did not impact the correlation between SA and GS. In other words, it suggests that not only gets score but also there was a possibility of intentional losing score.

6   Game Analysis Considering Play First and Play Second

Next, to tackle the problem not distinguishing between play first and play second mentioned in Sect. 4, we formulated a hypothesis that "the relation between SA and GS are different in play first and play second", and try to verify the hypothesis in the following paragraphs of the paper based on the game information database.

6.1   Method and Target Data

This method added the parameter of get score and lose score to the method described in Sect. 4.1.

Specifically, when we extracted the DFGS and shot accuracy for each collected game, we define the mean value of SA regarding all ends as Total Shot Accuracy (TSA), the mean value of SA regarding end for play first teams as Play first Shot Accuracy ($1stSA$), and the mean value of SA regarding an end for play second teams as Play second Shot Accuracy ($2ndSA$).

Next, we examined the correlation between DFGS and difference in SA[6]. Furthermore, these results were compared separately for each player gender.

As target data we used 93 games of Sochi Winter Olympic Games similarly to the data described in Sect. 4.2.

---

[6] Hereinafter, this is called Difference in Total Shot Accuracy ($DTSA$), Difference in Play first Shot Accuracy ($D1stSA$), Difference in Play second Shot Accuracy ($D2ndSA$).

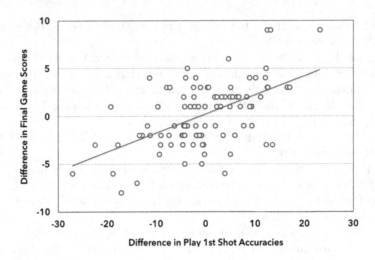

Fig. 13. Correlation between difference in play 1st shot accuracies vs. difference in final game scores [21].

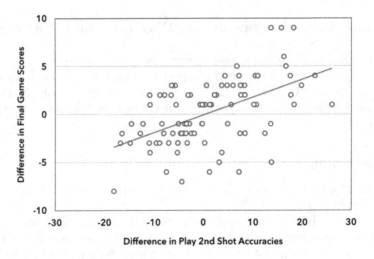

Fig. 14. Correlation between difference in play 2nd shot accuracies vs. difference in final game scores [21].

6.2   Result of Analysis

Here we describe the relation between SA and GS separately for play first and play second cases. Figure 13 shows a diagram representing a correlation between D1stSA and DFGS and regression line and Fig. 14 stands for a correlation between D2ndSA and DFGS.

In Figs. 13 and 14, the X axis shows each SA (D1stSA or D2ndSA) for each game and the Y axis represents the DFGS. Correlation for play first teams was 0.557 and for play second teams it was 0.530.

Therefore, it can be confirmed that the two differences in Figs. 13 and 14 have a positive correlation. These results are similar to that of the results in Sect. 4, in both play first and play second, the difference in each SA becomes larger as the DFGS is larger.

Next, we analyzed the correlation for male and female players using a similar technique. Table 2 shows the correlation between each difference in SA and DFGS separated by gender.

Table 2. Pearson's correlation between each difference in shot accuracy and difference in final game score separated by gender [21].

	All games	Men	Women
Total	0.670	0.634	0.707
Play first	0.557	0.564	0.545
Play second	0.530	0.532	0.547

As shown in Table 2, the correlation coefficient between DTSA and DFGS for men was 0.634 and for women was 0.707. In addition, the correlation coefficient when a team was in play first position for men was 0.564, for women it was 0.545 and when a team was in play second position for men it was 0.532, and for women it was 0.547.

Next, we carried out the *test for the hypothesis that several correlations are estimates of the same correlation* [22] to examine the Pearson's correlation between each difference in SA and if DFGS were statistically significant. As a result of the test, there were no significant differences between the three correlations (DTSA and DFGS, D1stSA and DFGS, and between D2ndSA and DFGS).

According to the above results, it dismissed the previously proposed hypothesis that "the relation between SA and GS are different in play first and play second". It means that there were no significant differences between correlations when teams were in play first or play second positions.

7 Discussion

In this section, we describe the discussion on analysis results in Sects. 5 and 6. By analysis considering get score and lose score, it was proven that get and lose score did not influence the relation between SA and GS for game information of world national top level.

Additionally, there were no significant differences between correlations when teams were in play first and play second positions in analysis of Sect. 6.

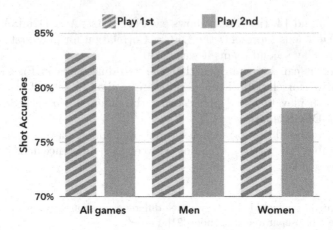

Fig. 15. Shot accuracy divided by gender and playing position [21].

We can propose the following reasons for these results. Firstly, game information for world national top level has sufficiently high SA. Secondly, the relation between SA and GS did not include the parameters relating to the starting position (play first or play second) and, getting/losing score. These results are not in contradiction with examination that the relation between SA and GS for world national top level is involved with the game result and it was influenced by selected tactics or strategies in Sect. 4. Therefore, to extract a characteristic in strategies of world national top level, we need to compare the result of similar analysis other than player level or consider the parameter other than SA.

Next, we carried out an analysis focusing on parameters other than SA to investigate influential parameters that relate to team strategies for world class.

Figure 15 shows 1stSA and 2ndSA in analysis subject separately by gender.

As Fig. 15 shows, there was a tendency that 1stSA were higher than 2ndSA through as the whole they matched. For men, the 1stSA was 84.26%, the 2ndSA was 82.17% and the difference between the play first and play second was 2.09 point. In the SA for women, the 1stSA was 81.84%, the 2ndSA was 78% and the difference between the play first and play second was 3.84 point. These results mean there is a difference between performing 1 to 2 shots per a game.

This suggests that the players playing in the second position performed more difficult shots than in play first, which may be related to shot option and its degree of difficulty.

Based on the above, we analyzed the data by focusing on how many of which types of shots were thrown using 8 games of a playoff in the championships.

Figures 16 and 17 show the ratio of each type of shot in play first and play second positions.

By comparing Fig. 16 with Fig. 17, the ratios of *takeout shots* were almost the same. However, ratios of *draw shots* were different between play first and play second. In particular, the ratio of *Come-around* shot which is one of the

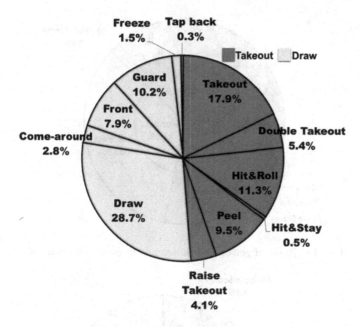

Fig. 16. Ratio of shots by types in play first position.

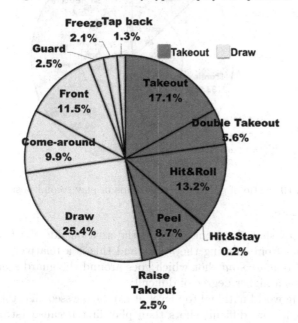

Fig. 17. Ratio of shots by types in play second position.

draws for play second was higher than in a play first. Additionally, the ratio of *Guard* shot for playing first was performed more often than in play second.

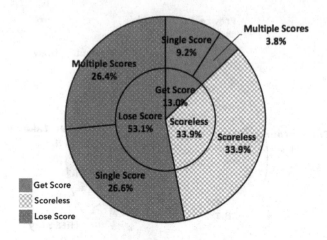

Fig. 18. Ratio of get or lose score ends in play first position.

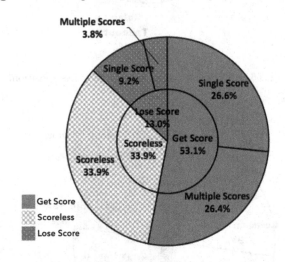

Fig. 19. Ratio of get or lose score ends in play second position.

In the *Guard* shot the stone stops in the area outside the *house* to block opponent stones from entering the *house* and this is a relatively easy shot. In contrast, the *Come-around* shot which goes around the guard stone and stops in the house has a higher degree of difficulty.

Therefore, in world national top level, it can be guessed that the play second team performed more difficult shots than play first because 1stSA are higher than 2ndSA. It can be guessed that the shot requested and its degree of difficulty differs depending on the starting position because the player has to perform a shot considering the state of one's own team or the match situation.

Next, we make an investigation into ratios of getting score ends, lose score ends, scoreless ends in play first and play second positions. Figures 18 and 19 show the ratio of get or lose score in playing first and play second positions.

As Fig. 18 shows, in play first, ratio of get score ends was 13.0% (get 1 score ends was 9.2%, get multiple scores was 3.8%), ratio of scoreless ends was 33.9%, ratio of lose score ends was 53.1% (lose 1 score ends was 26.6%, lose multiple scores was 26.4%). In play second, ratio of get score ends was 53.1% (get 1 score ends was 26.6%, get multiple scores was 26.4%), ratio of scoreless ends was 33.9%, ratio of lose score ends was 13.0% (lose 1 score ends was 9.2%, lose multiple scores was 3.8%).

It explains that the ratio of get score ends in play first was much greater than in play second because play second team has an advantage of performing the last stone in the end. Additionally, in play first, get 1 score is 5.4 points more than get multiple score ends. On the other hand, in play second, ratio of get 1 score ends is almost similar to get multiple scores.

Because of the above result, play first teams can be said to take tactics of minimizing damage by the opposite team, meanwhile, the opposite teams take tactics to gain multiple scores and increase difference in GS for play second position.

Therefore, in world national top level, it can be said that play first teams take tactics to strike the first blow for opponent and keep to a minimum lose score by performing more *Guard* shots, while play second teams aim to increase the score by performing the shots that go around the guard stones.

Thus, this supports the tendencies that the strategies/tactics taken by each team differ in play first and play second starting positions by investigating the ratio of shots by types and ratio of get or lose score.

In the near future, by analyzing the above parameters using a machine learning method, we plan to extract characteristics of team tactics in detail. In addition, we plan to extract information useful in tactical support by applying a Digital curling technology developed by Yamamoto et al. [23] and Ito et al. [24] which contains world national top level game with SA.

8   Conclusion

In this paper, we performed an analysis of game information from a number of curling game matches using *iCE*, a digital scorebook.

The result suggested that the difference in shot accuracies is related to the difference in the game scores. Also, we confirmed that this correlation in world class is lower than the Japanese national class. Furthermore, we analyzed the game information of outliers from tactical point of view. It was proven that the selected tactics and a contributing shot and pressure on the opponent team had an impact on the game result.

Next, we added a parameter of get/lose score and starting position to the above analysis, and carried out an analysis of the relation between shot accuracy and game score. The result confirmed that the correlation was lower for get scores, and there were no significant differences between the play first and play second. Thus, it confirmed that the relation between shot accuracy and game score did not contribute to game results in world national top class.

Furthermore, we discussed why it was not possible to confirm a significant difference and indicated a need for other influential parameters than shot accuracy. The result suggested that the ratio of shots by types and ratio of get or lose score relates to strategies in world class.

In the near future, we plan to record game information of world national top level and analyze it focusing on parameters other than shot accuracy (e.g. throwing number by type of shot) in detail. In addition, we will aim to propose techniques for strategies/tactics analysis considering strategic characteristics.

Acknowledgments. This work was supported by JSPS KAKENHI (grant number: 15H02797).

References

1. Bradley, L.J.: The sports science of curling. A practical review. J. Sports Sci. Medi. **8**, 495–500 (2009)
2. Yanagi, H., Miyakoshi, K., Nakajima, Y., Yamamoto, N.: Development of curling brush for measuring force exerted during sweeping. In: Proceedings of the 30 International Conference on Biomechanics in Sports, pp. 354–356 (2012)
3. Takahashi, S.: Support the Japan women 's curling national team by a trainer. J. Train. Sci. Exerc. Sport **23**(1), 7–12 (2011). (in Japanese)
4. Masui, F., Hirata, K., Otani, H., Yanagi, H., Ptaszynski, M.: Informatics to support tactics and strategies in curling. Int. J. Autom. Technol. **10**(2), 244–252 (2016)
5. Fujimura, A., Sugihara, K.: Quantitative evaluation of sport teamwork using generalized Voronoi diagrams. IEICE Trans. D **J87–D2**, 818–828 (2004)
6. Kagawa, M.: Effect of multimedia information on web pages in physical training class of university. J. Jpn. Soc. Educ. Technol. **29**, 37–40 (2006)
7. Ueno, H., Masui, F., Yanagi, H.: Development of a portable database system for supporting curling tactics. In: Proceedings of 25th National Conference of Japan Society of Training Science for Exercise and Sport (2012). (in Japanese)
8. Masui, F., Ueno, F., Yanagi, H., Ptaszynski, M.: Toward curling informatics digital scorebook development and game information analysis. In: Proceedings of 2015 IEEE Conference on Computer Intelligence and Games, pp. 481–488 (2015)
9. Hirata, K., Masui, F., Hiromu, O., Yanagi, H., Ptaszynski, M.: Support to strategies and tactics in curling sport utilizing game information database - analysis of characteristics of position based on shot scores. In: Proceedings of the 34th International Conference on Biomechanics in Sports, P0523433 (2016)
10. Shegelski, M.: The motion of a curling rock: analytical approach. Can. J. Phys. **78**, 857–864 (2000)
11. Denny, M.: Curling rock dynamics: towards a realistic model. Can. J. Phys. **80**, 1005–1014 (2002)
12. Maeno, N.: Dynamics and curl ratio of a curling stone. Sports Eng. **17**, 33–41 (2014)
13. Behm, D.G.: Periodized training program of the Canadian olympic curling team. J. Natl. Strength Cond. Assoc. Jpn. **16**(3), 40–47 (2009)

14. Tanaka, Y., Tsubota, H., Takeda, Y., Tsuji, T.: Analysis of human hand movements using a virtual curling system. In: Proceedings of Conference on Robotics and Mechatronics, 1A1-3F-E1 (2006). (in Japanese)
15. Igarashi, H., Ishihara, S. and Kimura, M.: A Study of policy-gradient methods in non-markov decision processes: curling game application. IEICE Technical report, NC2006-148, pp. 179–184 (2007). (in Japanese)
16. Ura, M., Endo, S., Miyazaki, S., Yasuda, T.: Curling game simulation and strategies evaluation. In: Proceedings of the Virtual Reality Society of Japan, Annual Conference, vol. 13, 2B3-5 (2007). (in Japanese)
17. Sung, G.P.: Curling analysis based on possession of the last stone per end. Procedia Eng. **60**, 391–396 (2013). 6th Asia Pacific Congress on Sports Technology
18. Howard, R.: Curl to Win: Expect Advice to Improve Your Game. HarperCollins Publishers Ltd., New York City (2009)
19. Coleman, G.: Introduction to Curling Strategy (English Edition). Amazon Services International Inc., Seattle (2014)
20. Otani, H., Masui, F., Hirara, K., Yanagi, H., Ptaszynski, M.: Analysis of curling team strategy and tactics using curling informatics. In: 4th International Congress on Sport Sciences Research and Technology Support (2016)
21. Otani, H., Masui, F., Yanagi, H., Ptaszynski, M.: Advances in curling game information analysis by considering starting position. In: 5th International Congress on Sport Sciences Research and Technology Support (2017)
22. Paul, S.R.: Test for the equality of several correlation coefficients*. Can. J. Stat. **17**(2), 217–227 (1989)
23. Yamamoto, M., Kato, S., Iizuka, H.: Digital curling strategy based on game tree search. In: Proceedings of IEEE-CIG 2015 (2015)
24. Ito, T., Kitasei, Y.: Proposal and implementation of digital curling. In: Proceedings of IEEE-CIG 2015 (2015)

Novel Approaches for Geometrical Model-Based Calculation of Human Body Segment Inertial Parameter Values

Arnold Baca[1]([⊠]), Michaela Hassmann[1], Philipp Kornfeind[1],
and Pelin Cizgin[2]

[1] Department of Biomechanics/Kinesiology and Computer Science in Sport,
University of Vienna, Vienna, Austria
arnold.baca@univie.ac.at
[2] Institute of Molecular Biotechnology, Vienna, Austria

Abstract. In human motion analysis, inverse dynamic solutions are used for the determination of joint reaction forces and net joint torques. This approach requires a full kinematic description, external forces and, most important, accurate anthropometric measures. For the estimation of human body segment parameter values, several methods have been proposed in literature throughout the last 120 years. The paper gives an overview of historical and contemporary methods with a specific focus on approaches based on geometrical models of the human body. Methods for (semi-)automated shape detection, segmentation and calculation of anthropometric dimensions are presented and compared. Body segment parameters of Hatze's hominoid model can be estimated applying image based or photogrammetric techniques. Results of an evaluation study on 6 subjects (3 male, 3 female) by comparing principal moments of inertia and total body masses are shown. The calculation of body segment inertial parameters from 3D surface scanning techniques has proven to be a fast and accurate method without exposing subjects to radiation. Future developments in application of mobile 3D scanning techniques can be expected to further ease handling and reduce costs.

Keywords: Anthropometry · Inverse dynamics · Human motion analysis

1 Introduction

Human movement can be described by numerous kinematic variables, such as displacements, velocities, accelerations and joint angles. In addition, kinetic data such as ground reaction forces are measured, as pure kinematic approaches are often not sufficient [1]. The prediction of joint reaction forces and net joint torques, which actually caused the movement, allows understanding forces acting on and within the human body. These forces are generally calculated indirectly using kinematic, kinetic and anthropometric data, which is called an inverse solution, a very powerful tool in motion analysis [2]. A reliable biomechanical link-segment model requires accurate estimation of human body segment parameter values (BSP). These parameters comprise volume, mass, location of center of mass, principal moments of inertia and location of the

© Springer Nature Switzerland AG 2019
J. Cabri et al. (Eds.): icSPORTS 2016/2017, CCIS 975, pp. 150–163, 2019.
https://doi.org/10.1007/978-3-030-14526-2_10

principal axes of inertia. BSP and their accurate estimation have been of great interest first in aeronautics and aerospace, later in clinical settings, ergonomics and sport. Studies have addressed the problem of accurate estimation of BSP [1] and shown the sensitivity of inverse dynamic solutions to BSP [3]. BSP are mostly validated by comparing calculated ground reaction forces based on BSP deviation with force plate data as the ground truth [4]. Different approaches for estimating BSP with a specific focus on recent developments towards easier applicability of geometrical models are summarized in this paper, which is an updated and extended version of [5].

2 An Overview of Methods

Several different approaches have been followed identifying individual BSP. We will differentiate between and describe statistical methods, methods based on medical imaging technologies, dynamic parameter estimation methods and geometrical models.

2.1 Statistical Methods

Regression equations incorporating whole body and/or segment anthropometric measurements were first derived from human cadaver studies by Braune and Fischer [6], Dempster [7], Clauser, McConville and Young [8], while Drillis and Contini [9] used water immersion and compound pendulum method on living humans. These equations provide simple and fast methods for BSP prediction and therefore they are still widely used, while several drawbacks to this method have been addressed. Prediction is based on data from a small number of elderly male cadavers, which may result in limited accuracy for different age and gender [10, 11]. Erdmann and Kowalczyk [12] propose a method for estimating volume, mass and location of center of mass of body segments using data from [8] and additional computed tomography (CT) scans. Based on regression equations developed by Erdmann [13] they divided the trunk into subparts consisting of tissues of different density.

2.2 Methods Based on Medical Imaging Technologies

Predictive models for BSP estimation based on in vivo human data involve the use of gamma ray scanning [14], dual energy X-ray absorptiometry (DEXA) [15, 16], computed tomography (CT) [17], magnetic resonance imaging (MRI) [18] and combinations of methods. Gamma ray scanning, DEXA and CT underlie criticism because of exposure to radiation [11], whereas in MRI no radiation is applied. In general, the use of medical imaging methods is limited due to relatively high costs and time consumption, even if they provide reliable and accurate BSP estimations directly on living subjects [11, 19].

2.3 Dynamic Parameter Estimation Methods

Recently, methods applying parameter fitting approaches based on kinematics and measured external forces have been published. Bonnet et al. [20] identify inertial parameters using optimal excitation motions and body postures and experimentally validated their proposed method with only one human subject. BSP identification considering robotics formalism is applied on the head complex, by firstly estimating mass and center of gravity from a static model and secondly estimating the moment of inertia from a dynamic model [21]. Son et al. [22] evaluate the feasibility of using a Biodex dynamometer for the estimation of inertial parameters. They suggest a method based on the dynamic equation of motion and an optimization technique. The latter two methods can determine inertial parameters for selected segments only.

2.4   Methods Based on Geometrical Models

Geometrical models map human body parts to segments described by simple regular geometric shapes. The dimensions of these shapes are defined by a number of anthropometric measurements according to the respective model. The most popular model is the Hanavan model [23] which requires only 25 anthropometric dimensions for the definition of all 15 body segments. To our knowledge, the most accurate mathematical model for the computational estimation of BSP is the "hominoid"

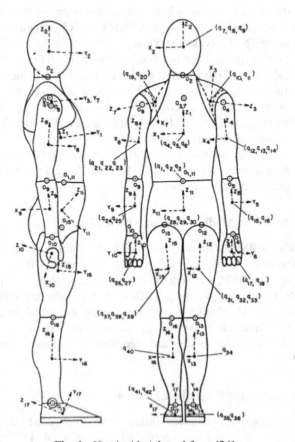

Fig. 1. Hominoid. Adapted from [24].

published by Hatze [24, 25]. The "hominoid" differentiates between male and female subjects concerning exomorphic and tissue density differences and takes into account age, segmental shape fluctuations and asymmetries in geometries of 17 segments (see Fig. 1). To this end, segments are sectioned into several geometric shapes, from which the volume can be estimated. As a result, 242 anthropometric input values are required, including height, diameter and circumference measurements. In addition, a non-uniform volume and density function are used [25]. However, the manual determination of the required 242 anthropometric dimensions takes about 60–80 min.

3   Automated Shape Detection of Human Body Segments

Even though geometric models incorporating a non-uniform density function like the hominoid enable a very accurate BSP estimation, their application in practice is rare. This is due to the high timely effort required for obtaining model parameters. In a clinical setup, for example, this is a relevant cost factor. In addition to safe and accurate methods, rapid availability of results and cost-effectiveness are of high importance.

In order to overcome this problem, image based or photogrammetric approaches may be utilized. Their application enables capturing 2D- or 3D-shape related data and calculating the geometric outlines of body segments without much effort. Different setups have been introduced. Microsoft Kinect based sensor systems have, for example, been applied by Clarkson, Choppin, Hart, Heller, and Wheat [26] and Clarkson, Wheat, Heller, and Choppin [27]. Bragança et al. [28] have compared anthropometric data collected using one particular Kinect body imaging system with manually measured data. Only few measurements were below a standardized allowable error. It was assumed that this was because of the long duration to acquire the data by the Kinect system. Peyer, Morris, and Seller [29], Stančić, Musić, and Zanchi [30], Sheets, Corazza, and Andriacchi [31] as well as Lu and Wang [32] made use of 3D scanners. Jafari Roodbandi et al. [33] compared anthropometric dimensions obtained by a modified 3D scanner fabricated in their study with direct anthropometric measures. The accuracy of the system was rated as acceptable.

3.1   Faster Estimation of Anthropometric Dimensions for the Hominoid

There have been several attempts to reduce the high effort in obtaining the anthropometric data required as input for Hatze's hominoid. Bogner [34] and Tscherne [35] developed regression equations and algorithms in order to predict some of the required dimensions from others.

Baca [36] introduced a method for calculating the required data applying image processing algorithms. Four different body configurations are recorded in order to determine the shapes of the 17 segments of the hominoid. Thin black ribbons are wrapped around selected segment boundaries in order to detect these boundaries in the recorded images with higher accuracy (Fig. 2). Baca compares his method to that based on manual measurements and reports differences below 5% in length, mass and volume and below 10% of principal moments of inertia of large segments. However, the method is still somewhat time consuming, because of the recording procedure.

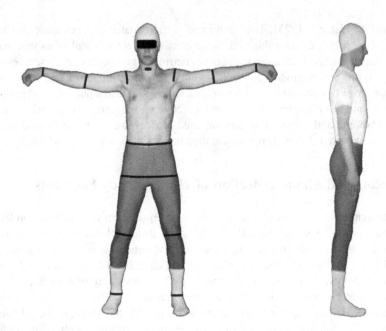

Fig. 2. Two of four recording positions for determination of anthropometric dimensions of hominoid model [36].

3.2   Application of Full Body 3D Scanners

The increasing performance of 3D scanners provides novel means for estimating anthropometric dimensions. A three-dimensional mesh of the human body surface can be obtained fast, accurate and reliable. From this, coordinates of measuring points defining anthropometric measures of interest may be determined. By combining these technologies and accurate mathematical segment models incorporating adequate geometric shapes and non-uniform density distributions not only accurate but, moreover, fast estimation BSP may be provided.

Three-dimensional body scanning technology (Vitus Smart XXL, Vitronic, Wiesbaden, Germany) has therefore been utilized for determining individual anthropometric dimensions of Hatze's hominoid model being used as input parameters for calculating subject specific BSP. The scanning device used allows capturing full body scans with an accuracy of ±1 mm. Figure 3 depicts an example of a 3D-scan. An automated approach for segmentation [37] and a semi-automated approach [38] have been pursued.

3.2.1   Automated Approach

In her master thesis, Schiffl [37] developed and evaluated a method for automatically identifying segment boundaries and segment volumes according to the 17-segment hominoid of Hatze. Her algorithms were based on 3D scans obtained from one scanning position. No ribbons were wrapped around segment boundaries nor were any markers attached to the subjects being scanned. It was possible to identify the 17 segments from the scan data. An exemplary result is shown in Fig. 4.

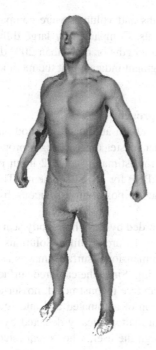

Fig. 3. 3D-scan from Vitus Smart XXL 3D body scanner.

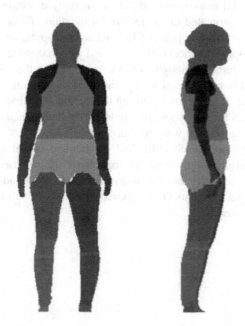

Fig. 4. Automated segmentation (adapted from Schiffl [37]).

Results for segment lengths and volumes were compared to those obtained from manual reference measurements. Comparatively large differences, such as more than 15% differences in upper arm lengths or more than 20% difference in the volumes of the thoracic and the pelvic segment indicate that the method is not accurate enough for practical applications.

3.2.2   Semi-automated Approach

In order to increase accuracy, a semi-automated method has therefore been developed and evaluated [38]. Within her master thesis, Cizgin proposed a procedure, which in total takes about 10–12 min for estimating all 242 input parameter values describing Hatze's model and from this BSP for all 17 segments. The approach combines automated calculation and interactive positioning of icons by the user and is therefore classified as semi-automated.

Whole body scans are recorded by the whole-body scanner (Vitus Smart XXL) and processed by the ScanWorX software (Human Solutions, Kaiserslautern, Germany). The software captures three-dimensional surface images as point clouds and saves the recorded data for later processing. Since the captured surface cloud point images are in sufficient detail and almost gap free reconstructed, no surface mesh procedures had to be implemented. A combination of automated and interactive measurements has been realized: Several landmarks are automatically detected by means of the software, the remaining are estimated through the user, who is requested to mark specific positions on the scan data.

The subject to be analysed has to wear thight fitting clothing, and a bathing cap to mask the hairs. 5 circular markers are attached to the body at certain reference positions in order to facilitate automated or interactive localization. These positions comprise right jaw joint, most protruding point of left and right scapula, left and right hip joint center. In the development process, it was found out that these reference positions cannot be detected accurately enough from the scan without the use of marker points. Subjects are recorded in two defined scan positions. The duration for one scan is about 12 s. Subjects have to try not to move during that period. The first posture is shown in Fig. 3. Since measures for the upper arm could not be determined from the respective scan, another recording posture was introduced (Fig. 5).

In the hominoid model, each individual geometrical model is assigned its own density [24, 36]. There are four direct anthropometric measurements required, which are used to derive the subcutaneous fat content at the hip and to adjust the densities of specific parts of certain segments. These measurements have still to be performed by the direct measuring method.

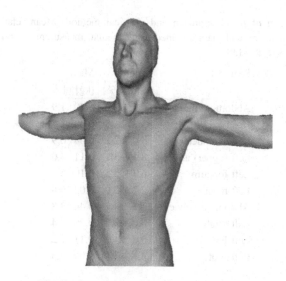

Fig. 5. Scanning position for posture 2 [38].

ScanWorX's module AnthroScan automatically detects almost all reference and landmark points defined in Hatze's hominoid model from the two scans. Users get a view of the three-dimensional point clouds recorded and the estimated landmark positions and can either confirm these positions or correct them interactively. The software has been extended and adapted, so that all 242 subject specific parameter values characterizing the hominoid model can now be determined. Figure 6 shows as an example the visualization of a virtual tape for taking the perimeters and length measures of the underarm and leg within the 3D scan image.

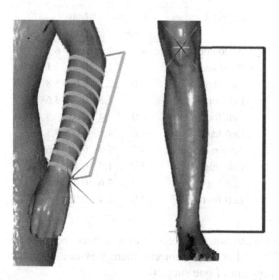

Fig. 6. Virtual tape for taking perimeters and length measures [5, 38].

Table 1. Comparison of novel approach and classical method: Mean relative and absolute differences between length and mass obtained using manual measurement and semi-automated approach for male subjects [38].

Segment	Length		Mass	
	[mm]	[%]	[kg]	[%]
Abdomino-thoracic	6.7	1.3	0.70	1.9
Head neck	3.3	1.5	0.09	2.7
Left shoulder	3.0	2.2	0.08	6.9
Left (upper) arm	8.3	3.1	0.11	4.0
Left forearm	6.7	2.5	0.10	5.3
Left hand	2.7	2.9	0.03	6.8
Abdomino-pelvic	11.3	4.2	0.44	3.8
Left thigh	10.0	3.2	0.20	2.4
Left leg	5.3	1.3	0.11	7.2
Left foot	4.3	1.8	0.04	6.3

In an evaluation study, the semi-automated approach was compared to the classical method based on manual measurements. 3 male (27.0 ± 2.6 yrs, 183.3 ± 4.5 cm, 81.7 ± 7.4 kg) and 3 female (25.7 ± 2.3 yrs, 169.7 ± 10.4 cm, 55.1 ± 2.2 kg) subjects were studied. Mean absolute and relative differences in segment lengths and masses are given in Tables 1 (male) and 2 (female), mean relative differences in principal moments of inertia in Tables 3 (male) and 4 (female).

Table 2. Comparison of novel approach and classical method: Mean relative and absolute differences between length and mass obtained using manual measurement and semi-automated approach for female subjects [38].

Segment	Length		Mass	
	[mm]	[%]	[kg]	[%]
Abdomino-thoracic	4.7	1.1	0.80	6.2
Head neck	2.3	1.1	0.12	2.1
Left shoulder	3.0	2.7	0.04	5.8
Left (upper) arm	3.7	1.3	0.05	3.6
Left forearm	6.0	2.4	0.01	0.9
Left hand	3.0	4.1	0.02	8.3
Abdomino-pelvic	4.3	1.9	0.17	1.6
Left thigh	5.3	1.7	0.15	2.2
Left leg	6.3	1.6	0.04	1.5
Left foot	5.0	2.4	0.05	7.6

Differences in the position of the center of mass were below 9 mm for all segments of all female subjects. For male subjects, there was one exception (14 mm for the abdomino-pelvic segment of one subject).

Table 3. Comparison of novel approach and classical method: Mean relative differences between principal moments of inertia obtained using manual measurement and semi-automated approach for male subjects [38].

Segment	Principal moments of inertia		
	x	y	z
	[%]	[%]	[%]
Abdomino-thoracic	5.1	5.7	5.9
Head neck	3.4	3.0	3.1
Left shoulder	7.7	7.7	13.4
Left (upper) arm	8.2	8.7	5.9
Left forearm	12.0	11.7	12.7
Left hand	10.6	16.7	15.8
Abdomino-pelvic	10.8	2.9	10.4
Left thigh	5.6	5.3	3.6
Left leg	2.6	2.6	5.4
Left foot	1.4	5.4	7.6

In general, both negative and positive deviations were observed. The largest differences were identified in principal moments of inertia of small segments, which typically have limited influence on the result of analyses of whole-body motions.

Table 4. Comparison of novel approach and classical method: Mean relative differences between principal moments of inertia obtained using manual measurement and semi-automated approach for female subjects [38].

Segment	Principal moments of inertia		
	x	y	z
	[%]	[%]	[%]
Abdomino-thoracic	9.5	9.5	11.3
Head neck	4.2	3.2	3.2
Left shoulder	4.8	18.3	7.9
Left (upper) arm	9.2	9.4	4.1
Left forearm	2.4	2.4	3.1
Left hand	11.0	25.2	19.6
Abdomino-pelvic	3.8	5.2	3.4
Left thigh	2.3	2.3	5.6
Left leg	6.6	6.9	2.0
Left foot	5.6	5.6	15.0

Total body masses have been determined by applying the novel approach and the classical method and adding the masses of the individual segments as well as by measuring this mass by using a scale. Results are given in Table 5.

Table 5. Comparison of total body masses for male (1–3) and female (4–6) subjects [38].

Subject	Classical	Scanner	Scale	Scale vs. classical	Scale vs. scanner
	[kg]	[kg]	[kg]	[%]	[%]
1	77.3	76.1	76.8	0.68	0.88
2	90.4	89.8	90.2	0.19	0.39
3	78.3	77.7	78.1	0.26	0.57
4	56.3	57.1	56.2	0.19	1.67
5	51.6	52.4	52.5	1.75	0.14
6	55.4	56.5	56.5	1.91	0.00

On average, this is a difference of 0.83% when comparing the classical method to and a difference of 0.61% when comparing the novel approach to the scale measurement.

The semi-automatic approach has shown to be promising for estimating BSP fast and accurate. It takes about 12 to 15 min to determine the required data for one subject. This is about 15–20% of the time required for the procedure based on manual measurements.

A general drawback of methods based on the particular 3D scanner used lies in the comparatively high costs and stationarity of the scanning device. It should, however, be possible substituting this specific instrument by scanners demanding lower costs (for example as described in Peyer, Morris, and Seller [29], given that a similar scan resolution may be obtained. Redlarski et al. [39] calculated human body surface area using hand-held Artec 3D Eva scanner. Centre of gravity estimation from 3D surface scans with a low-cost, hand-held mobile Sense 3D scanner was presented by Hassmann et al. [40].

4   Conclusion

The accurate BSP estimation requires appropriate geometric body segment models combined with a non-uniform density function. The large number of anthropometric dimensions needed for the definition of the geometric shapes leads to time-consuming procedures when carried out manually. Three-dimensional whole body scanning technology can reduce time for data collection significantly, as subjects have to maintain the recording position for only a few seconds. The semi-automated approach as described decreases the time for calculation of body segment parameters to some minutes. The validation proves reasonable accuracy of 3D body scanning compared to the manual method.

References

1. Cahouët, V., Martin, L., Amarantini, D.: Static optimal estimation of joint accelerations for inverse dynamics problem solution. J. Biomech. **35**(11), 1507–1513 (2002)
2. Winter, D.: Biomechanics and Motor Control of Human Movement, 4th edn. Wiley, New Jersey (2009)
3. Rao, G., Amarantini, D., Berton, E., Favier, D.: Influence of body segments' parameters estimation models on inverse dynamics solutions during gait. J. Biomech. **39**(8), 1531–1536 (2006)
4. Futamure, S., Bonnet, V., Dumas, R., Venture, G.: A sensitivity analysis method for the body segment inertial parameters based on ground reaction and joint moment regressor matrices. J. Biomech. **64**, 85–92 (2017)
5. Cizgin, P., Kornfeind, P., Haßmann, M., Baca, A.: Advancements of methods for fast and accurate estimation of human body segment parameter values. In: Proceedings of the 5th International Congress on Sport Sciences Research and Technology Support, vol. 1, pp. 69–74. icSPORTS. https://doi.org/10.5220/0006439400690074
6. Braune, W., Fischer, O.: Der Körperschwerpunkt Deutscher Infanteristen. ATI 138 452. National Technical Information Service, Leipzig (1889)
7. Dempster, W.T.: Space requirements for the seated operator. Wright Air Development Center WADC. Technical report TR-55-159. Wright-Patterson Air Force Base, Dayton (1955)
8. Clauser, C.E., McConville, J.T., Young, J.W.: Weight, volume and center of mass of segments of the human body. AMRL Technical report. Wright-Patterson Air Force Base, Dayton (1969)
9. Drillis, R., Contini, R.: Body Segment Parameters. Report No. 1166-03. Office of Vocational Rehabilitation, New York (1966)
10. Nigg, B.M., Herzog, W.: Biomechanics of the Muskulo-Skeletal System, 2nd edn. Wiley, Chichester (1999)
11. Durkin, J.L.: Measurement and estimation of human body segment parameters. In: Hong, Y., Bartlett, R. (eds.) Routledge Handbook of Biomechanics and Human Movement Science, pp. 197–213. Routledge, London (2008)
12. Erdmann, W.S., Kowalczyk, R.: A personalized method for estimating centre of mass location of the whole body based on differentiation of tissues of a multi-divided trunk. J. Biomech. **48**(1), 65–67 (2015)
13. Erdmann, W.S.: Geometric and inertial data of the trunk in adult males. J. Biomech. **30**(7), 679–688 (1997)
14. Zatsiorsky, V., Seluyanov, V., Chugunova, L.: In vivo body segment inertial parameter determination using a gamma-scanner method. In: Berme, N., Cappozzo, A. (eds.) Biomechanics of Human Movement: Applications in Rehabilitation, Sports and Ergonomics, pp. 186–202. Bertec, Worthington (1990)
15. Durkin, J.L., Dowling, J.J., Andrews, D.M.: The measurement of body segment inertial parameters using dual energy X-ray absorptiometry. J. Biomech. **35**(12), 1575–1580 (2002)
16. Wicke, J., Dumas, G.A., Costigan, P.A.: Trunk density profile estimates from dual X-ray absorptiometry. J. Biomech. **41**(4), 861–867 (2007)
17. Ackland, T., Henson, P., Bailey, D.: The uniform density assumption: its effect upon the estimation of body segment inertial parameters. Int. J. Sports Biomech. **4**(2), 146–155 (1988)
18. Cheng, C.-K., Chen, H.-H., Chen, C.-S., Lee, C.-L., Chen, C.-Y.: Segment inertial properties of Chinese adults determined from magnetic resonance imaging. Clin. Biomech. **15**(8), 559–566 (2000)

19. Rossi, M., Lyttle, A., El-Sallam, A., Benjanuvatra, N., Blanksby, B.: Body segment inertial parameters of elite swimmers using DXA and indirect methods. J. Sports Sci. Med. **12**(4), 761–775 (2013)

20. Bonnet, V., Fraisse, P., Crosnier, A., Gautier, M., González, A., Venture, G.: Optimal exciting dance for identifying inertial parameters of an anthropomorphic structure. IEEE Trans. Rob. **32**(4), 1–14 (2016)

21. Díaz-Rodríguez, M., Valera, A., Page, A., Besa, A., Mata, V.: Dynamic parameter identification of subject-specific body segment parameters using robotics formalism: case study head complex. J. Biomech. Eng. **138**(5), 051009 (2016)

22. Son, J., Ryu, J., Kim, J., Kim, Y.: Determination of inertial parameters using a dynamometer. Bio-Med. Mater. Eng. **24**(6), 2447–2455 (2014)

23. Hanavan, E.P.: A mathematical model of the human body. No. AFIT-GA-PHYS-64-3 Wright-Patterson Air Force Base, Dayton (1964)

24. Hatze, H.: A model for the computational determination of parameter values of anthropomorphic segments. CSIR Technical report TWISK 79, Pretoria (1979)

25. Hatze, H.: A mathematical model for the computational determination of parameter values of anthropomorphic segments. J. Biomech. **13**(10), 833–843 (1980)

26. Clarkson, S., Choppin, S., Hart, J., Heller, B., Wheat, J.: Calculating body segment inertia parameters from a single rapid scan using the Microsoft Kinect. In: Proceedings of 3rd International Conference on 3D Body Scanning Technologies, Lugano, Switzerland, 16–17 October (2012)

27. Clarkson, S., Wheat, J., Heller, B., Choppin, S.: Assessment of a Microsoft Kinect-based 3D scanning system for taking body segment girth measurements: a comparison to ISAK and ISO standards. J. Sports Sci. **34**(11), 1006–1014 (2016)

28. Bragança, S., Arezes, P., Carvalho, M., Ashdown, S.P., Xu, B., Castellucci, I.: Validation study of a Kinect based body imaging system. Work **57**(1), 9–21 (2017)

29. Peyer, K.E., Morris, M., Sellers, W.I.: Subject-specific body segment parameter estimation using 3D photogrammetry with multiple cameras. PeerJ **3**, e381 (2015). https://doi.org/10.7717/peerj.831

30. Stančić, I., Musić, J., Zanchi, V.: Improved structured light 3D scanner with application to anthropometric parameter estimation. Measurement **46**(1), 716–726 (2013)

31. Sheets, A.L., Corazza, S., Andriacchi, T.P.: An automated image-based method of 3D subject-specific body segment parameter estimation for kinetic analyses of rapid movements. J. Biomech. Eng. **132**(1), 011004 (2010)

32. Lu, J.-M., Wang, M.-J.J.: Automated anthropometric data collection using 3D whole body scanners. Expert Syst. Appl. **35**, 407–414 (2008)

33. Jafari Roodbandi, A.S., Naderi, H., Hashenmi-Nejad, N., Choobineh, A., Baneshi, M.R., Feyzi, V.: Technical report on the modification of 3-dimensional non-contact human body laser scanner for the measurement of anthropometric dimensions: verification of its accuracy and precision. J. Lasers Med. Sci. **8**(1), 22–28 (2017)

34. Bogner, M.: Regressionsanalyse anthropometrischer Daten zur Abschätzung von Segmentkonturdimensionen. Master thesis, University of Vienna (1992)

35. Tscherne, B.: Funktionsanpassungsalgorithmen für Datensequenzen anthropometrischer Dimensionen. Master thesis, University of Vienna (2001)

36. Baca, A.: Precise determination of anthropometric dimensions by means of image processing methods for estimating human body segment parameter values. J. Biomech. **29**(4), 563–567 (1996)

37. Schiffl, K.: Bestimmung von Hominoidsegmenten aus 3D-Bodyscannerdaten. Master thesis, Technical University Vienna (2011)

38. Cizgin, P.: Automatisierte Bestimmung anthropometrischer Segmentparameter des Hominoidmodells von Hatze mittels 3D-Laserscantechnologie. Master thesis, Medical University Vienna (2013)
39. Redlarski, G., Krawczuk, M., Palkowski, A.: Application of 3D whole body scanning in research on human body surface area. In: Book of Abstracts 3DBODY.TECH 2017 8th International Conference and Exhibition on 3D Body Scanning and Processing Technologies, Montreal, Canada, 11–12 October 2017
40. Hassmann, M., Markl, R., Friedl, N., Friedl, C., Krach, W.: Aerodynamics, EMG and 3D joint angles of different flight configurations of ATOS hang glider and pilot. A case study. In: Czaplicki, A., Wychowański, M., Wit, A. (eds.) International Conference of the Polish Society of Biomechanics 2016, pp. 105–106. Biała Podlaska, Polen (2016)

Computation of Optimal Release Parameters of Jump Shots in Basketball

Yuki Inaba$^{(\boxtimes)}$, Noriko Hakamada, and Munenori Murata

Department of Sport Science, Japan Institute of Sport Sciences,
3-15-1 Nishigaoka, Kita-ku, Tokyo, Japan
yuki.inaba@jpnsport.go.jp

Abstract. The purpose of this study was to establish the computational method to decide optimal release parameters by assessing the influence of selection of release parameters on the success rate of jump shots. The shooting performances from the free-throw (FT) and three-point (3P) lines of ten male collegiate basketball players were recorded using three-dimensional motion analysis system. The release parameters including release height, speed, angle, and spin rate were computed using the obtained positional data of the basketball. The resultant trajectory with selected release parameters were simulated using the equation of motion considering the influences of air drag and lift forces in the air. This enabled us to accurately investigate the influence of selection and variability of release parameters on the resultant trajectory, or the success rate. It ultimately resulted in computing optimal release parameters considering the actual influences on the success rate. In FT shots, decreasing magnitude of release speed and minimizing variability in release speed with larger margin for error for release speed contributed to higher success rate. For 3P shots, selecting release parameters that maximize margin for error for both release speed and release angle contributed to higher success rate since accurately grading the release speed was more difficult in shots from larger distance. Additionally, it was found that spin rate also does influence the trajectory of the ball in air. Therefore, it was concluded that when computing optimal release parameters, taking the influence of air drag and lift forces possibly caused by the spin of the ball into consideration is necessary since otherwise the relation between release parameters and resultant trajectory would be erroneous.

Keywords: Margin for error · Release parameters · Basketball

1 Introduction

Enhancing the successful shot percentages is critical for winning a basketball game. In particular, jump shots have been reported to be the most effective and frequently used shooting styles in a basketball game [1]. Thus, understanding the "better jump shots mechanics" which increases the successful shot percentages is essential for many basketball players and coaches.

Identifying a common and single good shooting motion which results in best successful shot percentages for every player is difficult since a number of possible combinations of joint motion exist for "a shooting motion" and players have different

© Springer Nature Switzerland AG 2019
J. Cabri et al. (Eds.): icSPORTS 2016/2017, CCIS 975, pp. 164–175, 2019.
https://doi.org/10.1007/978-3-030-14526-2_11

anthropometric characteristics. On the other hand, possible combinations of release parameters with higher successful shot percentages can be identified relatively easily since a ball trajectory after it is released is determined based on the release parameters. In particular, a ball trajectory with higher success rate can be defined from the number or range of possible successful trajectories from a certain release position. The number or range of possible successful trajectories is defined as a margin for error for the trajectories [2]. There are multiple successful paths for a ball successfully passing through the basket since the diameter of the basketball ring (0.45 m) is about the twice the diameter of the basketball (0.25 m). This means that selecting release parameters that increase the margin for error can be one of the factors which enhance the shooting success rate and can be one of the criteria to determine the optimal release parameters.

The range of successful paths is influenced by the entry angle of the ball into the basket ring (θ_e) since higher entry angles provide larger area for the successful paths of a ball passing through the basket [2]. The entry angle of the ball into the basket ring depends on release parameters such as the release speed, release angle, and release height based on the parabolic motion of the ball. In particular, previous studies have investigated the influences of selection of release angle and speed with a fixed release height [2, 3]. At a greater release angle, which accompanies a greater entry angle, the range of speed for a successful trajectory becomes larger. The range of release speeds with successful results at a selected release angle is called the margin for error for the speed. Thus, it can be assumed that increasing release angle to achieve a larger margin for error for the speed can be one possible strategy to increase the success rate. However, if the strategy to increase the release angle is selected, a higher release speed is required at the same time, which can negatively influence the consistency and accuracy of the movement [1]; lower release velocities accompany decreased movement variabilities [4]. In addition to that, a margin for error for the angle must be taken into consideration.

This trade-off between the release angle and the release speed was solved by the concept of "minimum-speed angle" [2]. Since the ratio of the margin for error for the speed to the release speed is very small compared to the release angle, and smaller release speed is advantageous, minimizing the release speed was used as the criteria to choose the optimal combination of the release parameters. Thus, the "minimum-speed angle" was regarded as the optimal release angle in theory [1]. Nevertheless, actual selection of release parameters by players during performing jump shots and those influences on the success rate have not been investigated. Thus, in this study, through investigating the relation between selected release parameters and those variabilities with shot results, definition of "optimal release parameters" were reconsidered.

In addition to the release angle and release speed, numerical analysis has suggested that having backspin and increasing the spin rate to about 3 rotations per second increase the possibility that free-throw shots are made [5–8]. In these studies, the main influence of back spin was not on the trajectory in air, but rather the behavior of the ball upon collision with the ring or backboard. In fact, these studies neglected the influences of the drag force and lift force in air, and some studies reported that the air resistance is negligible and does not have a significant effect on the trajectory of a ball [9]. However, there is a study [2] that implied that air resistance does have an effect on the trajectory though it is almost negligible. Therefore, in our study, effects of spin and air resistance on the ball trajectory was examined by analyzing the entire trajectory of the ball from release to arrival at the basket since the selection of the release parameters can be influenced if they affect the trajectories. Thus, the influences of the spin rate on the trajectory and the combination of the release angle and release speed were also investigated by simulating the ball trajectory at different ball spin rates.

2 Methods

2.1 Experimental Design

Ten male collegiate basketball players (height: 1.86 ± 0.07 m, body mass: 82.1 ± 7.4 kg, age: 22 ± 1 years-old, years of experience in basketball: 13 ± 3 years, mean $\pm$ standard deviation (SD)) participated in this study. They belong to a collegiate basketball team in the Japanese Kanto College Basketball Division 1 League. Three of them were selected to play for Japanese National Basketball Teams for the World University Games. Written informed consent to participate in the study was obtained from all participants after informing them of the purpose of this study and explaining the procedure and possible risks of the study. The study protocol was approved by the Human Subjects Committee of the Japan Institute of Sports Sciences.

The participants attempted 100 jump shots in total after a sufficient warm-up. Fifty shots were from the free-throw line (FT: 4.23 m away from the center of the ring in the horizontal direction). Another 50 shots were from the three-point line (3P: 6.75 m away from the center of the ring in the horizontal direction). Jump shots were attempted in a game-like situation, or after receiving a pass from an experienced basketball player positioned under the basketball goal ring. Participants were told to "perform a quick shot released at high position as you do in the game". A short break after each set of 25 shots was taken.

2.2 Data Collection

A three-dimensional motion analysis system using 20 cameras operating at 500 Hz (VICON MX series, Vicon Motion Systems Ltd., Oxford, UK) was used to track the position of the marks attached to the participants and a basketball. Forty-eight reflective markers were attached to the whole body of the participants. Nine to eleven reflective marks were randomly attached to the surface of the basketball.

2.3 Data Processing

Data processing was conducted in mainly three parts (Detail is shown in [10]). First, ball trajectories and spin rate were computed using the obtained marker positions of the marks attached to the ball's surface. Based on the equation of sphere, or the relation between the radius of the ball and the surface marks position, the position of the center of the ball was determined through optimization to minimize the least squares deviation. Secondly, based on the computed ball trajectories and spin rate, release parameters were estimated by optimization by a genetic algorithm to minimize the least-squares deviation between the calculated and actual (raw) trajectories. Since it has been reported that there is a significant influence of air drag to the trajectory [2], the equation of motion for the ball in air [11] was formulated as follows:

$$\ddot{r}_{ball} = a_D + a_N + a_G$$

where $\ddot{r}_{ball}$ is the acceleration of the ball, a_D is the acceleration by drag force, a_N is the acceleration by lift force, and a_G is the gravitational acceleration. Lastly, successful combinations of a release angle, a release speed, a spin rate, and a release height were estimated by simulating the trajectory of the ball at the given combinations of the release parameters. Using the equation of motion for the ball in air with the estimated coefficient of drag force and lift force, ball trajectories were recalculated for various combinations of the release angle and the release speed with the mean release height, horizontal distance from the ring center, spin rate. They were computed by solving the equation of motion using a fourth order Runge–Kutta algorithm. A shot was judged based on the arrival position of the ball when it reached the height of the goal ring (3.05 m) if it can be regarded as successful or not. The criteria for the successful was either "swish" where it could go through the ring without touching the rim (Fig. 1 green) or "barely touching the rim" which added the 50 mm margin to the swish criteria (Fig. 1 blue). Margin for error for the release speed and release angle, minimum-speed angle (traditional) were calculated as defined by Brancazio [2] and new minimum-speed angle was computed by calculating the possible minimum value of the release speed by approximating the successful combination area with the second order polynomial equation.

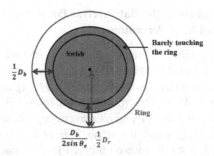

Fig. 1. The criteria for judging success (green: swish, blue: barely touching the ring, and white: missed). (Color figure online)

2.4 Statistics

A Pearson correlation coefficient was used to establish relationships between the success rate and the horizontal distance from the ring center, release parameters, and margins for errors. The level of significance was set at $p < 0.05$.

3 Results

3.1 Influence of the Drag and Lift Forces

The ball trajectory data was deviated in a great amount from the estimated trajectory based on the equation of parabolic motion using the initial velocity of the ball without considering the air drag and lift forces (Fig. 2). On the other hand, when the trajectory was estimated using the equation of motion with considering the drag and lift forces, the deviation was little.

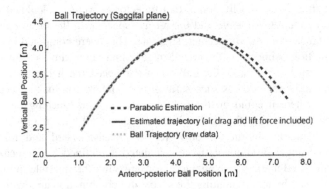

Fig. 2. The trajectory of the ball with different computation methods.

3.2 The Release Parameters, the Ball Arrival Positions, and the Successful Shot Percentages

The successful shot percentages, the release parameters (the release height, speed, and angle), and spin rate for FT (Table 1) and 3P (Table 2) were computed. The successful shot percentages for FT ranged from 64% (player 5) to 94% (player 1), and those for 3P ranged from 34% (player 4) to 72% (player 1 and player 3). The successful shot percentages for 3P were lower than FT in all players. Significant correlations between the successful shot percentages and the release height ($r = 0.82$, $p < 0.05$) and the release speed ($r = -0.63$, $p < 0.05$) were observed for FT shots. A significant correlation was found between the release speed and the SD of release speed ($r = 0.69$, $p < 0.05$). On the other hand, no significant correlations were observed between the successful shot percentages and the release parameters for 3P shots. The mean spin rates for FT and 3P were 132 ± 12 rpm and 128 ± 14 rpm, respectively. The spin rates did not have significant relationship between the successful percentages of the shots.

The mean and SD of the ball arrival positions (distances from the ring center and absolute distances from the ring center) for the FT shots and the 3P shots (Table 3) were computed. When an anteroposterior ball arrival position is over the ring center, it takes a positive value, and when it is short of the ring center, it takes a negative value. When a mediolateral ball arrival position is on the left side of the ring center in the player's view, it takes a positive value, and when it is on the right side, it takes a negative value. Significant correlations between the successful shot percentage and the SD of the anteroposterior distance of arrival position of the ball from the ring center for 50 FT shots and the SD of the absolute anteroposterior distance of arrival position of the ball from the ring center for 50 FT shots was observed. Also, significant correlations between the successful shot percentage and the mean distance of the arrival position from the ring in the anteroposterior and mediolateral directions, and SD of the anteroposterior distance of arrival position of the ball from the ring center for 50 3P shots were observed. In the FT shots, the difference of the anteroposterior arrival positions between the players with the highest and lowest success rate was smaller compared to the 3P shots (Fig. 3). However, it was obvious that Player 5 had greater variability in anteroposterior arrival positions than Player 1. On the other hand, the variability in anteroposterior arrival positions in 3P shots between the players with the highest and the lowest success rate were not as different as FT shots when compared with those in FT shots.

Table 1. Successful shot percentages and release and ball parameters for FT shots (*: $p < 0.05$).

Subject ID	Success rate 【%】	Rel. height 【m】		Rel. speed 【m/s】		Rel. angle 【deg】		Spin rate 【rpm】	
		Mean	SD	Mean	SD	Mean	SD	Mean	SD
1	94	2.77	0.01	6.72	0.07	44.1	1.3	148	7
2	90	2.53	0.01	6.83	0.07	47.4	1.0	136	5
3	88	2.71	0.02	6.85	0.09	44.5	1.6	118	7
4	84	2.58	0.02	6.83	0.09	47.6	1.7	128	7
5	64	2.42	0.01	6.97	0.09	46.6	1.3	141	7
6	92	2.71	0.01	6.85	0.10	47.6	1.3	132	7
7	82	2.62	0.01	6.81	0.06	45.6	1.1	133	5
8	84	2.51	0.02	6.83	0.07	47.2	1.1	148	7
9	92	2.71	0.03	6.90	0.10	50.4	1.4	114	8
10	78	2.45	0.03	7.07	0.10	49.9	1.0	118	7
Mean	85	2.60	0.02	6.86	0.08	47.1	1.3	132	7
SD	9	0.12	0.01	0.09	0.01	2.0	0.2	12	1
r	1	**0.82***	0.01	**−0.63***	−0.17	−0.07	0.15	−0.12	−0.17

Table 2. Successful shot percentages and release and ball parameters for 3P shots (*: $p < 0.05$).

Subject ID	Success rate 【%】	Rel. height 【m】		Rel. speed 【m/s】		Rel. angle 【deg】		Spin rate 【rpm】	
		Mean	SD	Mean	SD	Mean	SD	Mean	SD
1	72	2.59	0.01	8.61	0.07	46.1	1.3	145	8
2	66	2.49	0.02	8.43	0.07	46.8	1.2	145	6
3	72	2.67	0.01	8.51	0.07	42.4	1.3	125	10
4	34	2.33	0.02	8.75	0.08	50.4	1.5	111	9
5	54	2.41	0.01	8.57	0.06	45.3	1.3	139	7
6	68	2.69	0.01	8.56	0.11	49.5	1.7	125	6
7	52	2.62	0.02	8.46	0.07	44.5	0.8	133	7
8	62	2.59	0.01	8.32	0.10	44.1	1.2	133	10
9	71	2.63	0.03	8.69	0.07	50.6	1.3	109	13

(*continued*)

Table 2. *(continued)*

Subject ID	Success rate 【%】	Rel. height 【m】		Rel. speed 【m/s】		Rel. angle 【deg】		Spin rate 【rpm】	
		Mean	SD	Mean	SD	Mean	SD	Mean	SD
10	67	2.38	0.01	8.68	0.06	48.9	1.1	111	7
Mean	62	2.54	0.02	8.56	0.08	46.9	1.3	128	8
SD	12	0.13	0.01	0.13	0.01	2.9	0.2	14	2
r	1	0.58	0.10	−0.19	0.02	−0.15	−0.08	0.12	0.18

Table 3. Successful shot percentages and ball arrival positions for FT and 3P shots (*: $p < 0.05$).

		Success rate 【%】	Distance from ring center in 50 shots 【cm】				Absolute distance from ring center in 50 shots 【cm】			
			Anteroposterior		Mediolateral		Anteroposterior		Mediolateral	
			Mean	SD	Mean	SD	Mean	SD	Mean	SD
FT	Mean	85	5.5	9.2	0.7	6.4	9.0	6.6	5.5	4.0
	SD	9	4.2	1.5	2.5	1.0	2.7	1.5	0.8	0.6
	r	1	−0.46	−0.68*	0.34	−0.45	−0.56	−0.75*	−0.39	−0.30
3P	Mean	62	5.2	10.3	0.6	9.5	9.4	7.4	7.6	6.3
	SD	12	5.9	1.5	3.9	1.6	4.2	1.8	2.0	1.4
	r	1	−0.64*	−0.12	−0.16	−0.49	−0.59	−0.50	−0.63*	−0.65*

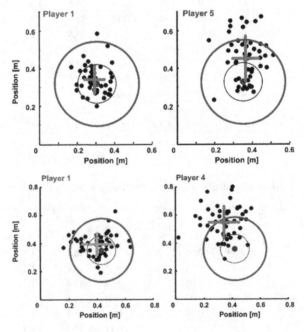

Fig. 3. The arrival positions of the ball of the 50 FT shots (Top) and 3P shots (bottom) of the player with the highest and the lowest success rate. Mean is the intersection between two blue lines which show the SD of the arrival positions in the anteroposterior and mediolateral directions. (Color figure online)

3.3 Comparison of the Selected and Theoretical Optimal Release Parameters

The actual selected combination of the release angle, the release speed, and the release height were compared with the theoretical successful combination of those parameters for player 1 with the highest successful percentages in the FT shots and player 5 with the lowest percentages (Fig. 4). The area of the successful combinations of release speed and release angle were larger for Player 1 than Player 5.

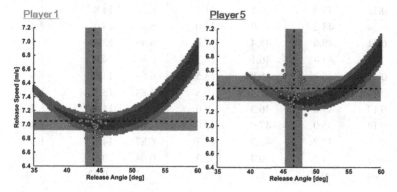

Fig. 4. Comparison of the selected (red) and theoretical combination of the release angle and the release speed (green: swish, blue: barely touching the ring) for the FT shots of the player 1 with the highest successful percentages and the player 5 with the lowest successful percentages. (Color figure online)

Also, the margin for error (ME) for the release speed at the mean selected release angle, traditional and new minimum-speed angle, ME for the release speed at minimum-speed angle, ME for the release angle at the mean selected release speed, optimal release speed which maximize the ME for release angle, ME for release angle at the optimal release speed, and combined ME were computed for FT (Table 4). ME for release speed at the actual mean release angle was greater in Player 1 (0.13 m/s) than Player 5 (0.11 m/s). ME for release speed and ME for release angle at optimal release speed had significant correlation with the successful shot percentages ($p < 0.05$). New minimum speed angles were smaller than traditional ones except FT shot condition of player 10.

The actual selected combination of the release angle, the release speed, and the release height were compared with the theoretical successful combination of those parameters for player 1 with the highest successful percentages in the 3P shots and player 4 with the lowest percentages (Fig. 5). Player 4 selected the larger release angle and release speed than optimal ones while Player 1 selected the release angle and release speed closer to the calculated optimal ones (Table 5).

Table 4. Margin for error for release speed and angle at the selected release parameters and the optimal condition for FT shots.

ID	Selected ME for rel. speed 【m/s】	Traditional minimum speed angle 【deg】	New minimum speed angle 【deg】	Selected ME for Rel. angle 【deg】	Optimal rel. speed 【m/s】	ME for rel. angle at optimal rel. speed 【deg】	Combined ME 【m/s deg】
1	**0.13**	**46.9**	**45.7**	**12.8**	**6.76**	**15.3**	**1.7**
2	0.14	48.6	47.3	10.8	6.88	13.8	1.5
3	0.13	47.3	46.1	11.5	6.82	14.8	1.5
4	0.14	48.2	47.0	14.0	6.83	14.0	2.0
5	**0.11**	**49.6**	**48.4**	**7.8**	**6.93**	**13.0**	**0.9**
6	0.15	47.4	46.1	14.3	6.86	14.8	2.1
7	0.12	48.1	46.8	13.5	6.84	14.3	1.6
8	0.14	48.5	47.4	10.8	6.88	13.8	1.5
9	0.17	47.6	46.3	9.0	6.86	14.8	1.5
10	0.14	45.0	47.9	13.0	7.07	13.0	1.8
Mean	0.14	47.7	46.9	11.7	6.87	14.1	1.6
SD	0.02	1.2	0.9	2.2	0.08	0.8	0.3
r	**0.64**	−0.30	**−0.87**	0.40	−0.57	**0.82**	0.61

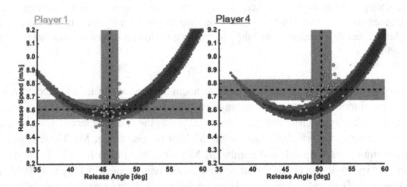

Fig. 5. Comparison of the selected (red) and theoretical combination of the release angle and the release speed (green: swish, blue: barely touching the ring) for the 3P shots of the player 1 with the highest successful percentages and the player 4 with the lowest successful percentages (revised from [10]). (Color figure online)

3.4   Influence of Spin Rate on the Theoretical Optimal Combination

The combination of the release angle and the release speed alternated by changing the spin rate (Fig. 6). For the selected release angles, the corresponding release speeds resulting in successful trajectories were lower for the higher spin rate condition (145 RPM) than the lower spin rate condition (109 RPM). New minimum speed angles and the release speeds with the largest margin for error for release angle were also lower at the higher spin rate condition.

Table 5. Margin for error for release speed and angle at the selected release parameters and the optimal condition for 3P shots.

ID	Selected ME for rel. speed 【m/s】	Traditional minimum speed angle 【deg】	New minimum speed angle 【deg】	Selected ME for rel. angle 【deg】	Optimal Rel. speed 【m/s】	ME for rel. angle at optimal rel. speed 【deg】	Combined ME 【m/s deg】
1	**0.12**	**47.0**	**45.4**	**11.3**	**8.62**	**12.0**	**1.3**
2	0.12	47.6	45.8	8.0	8.49	11.8	1.0
3	0.10	46.7	45.1	12.3	8.51	12.3	1.2
4	**0.14**	**48.4**	**46.8**	**4.5**	**8.63**	**11.5**	**0.6**
5	0.10	48.0	46.6	11.5	8.58	11.8	1.1
6	0.15	46.7	45.2	7.5	8.51	12.5	1.1
7	0.11	47.0	45.5	11.3	8.49	12.3	1.2
8	0.12	46.9	45.4	8.8	8.38	12.5	1.0
9	0.15	47.1	45.7	7.3	8.63	12.3	1.1
10	0.13	48.2	46.6	11.0	8.69	11.3	1.4
Mean	0.12	47.4	45.8	9.3	8.55	12.0	1.1
SD	0.02	0.6	0.6	2.5	0.09	0.4	0.2
r	0.00	−0.60	0.58	0.45	−0.06	0.35	**0.68**

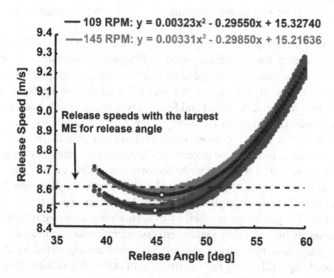

Fig. 6. Comparison of the successful combinations of release parameters of conditions with different spin rate (blue & gray 109 RPM, red and green 145 RPM). (Color figure online)

4 Discussion

The purpose of this study was to establish the computational method of optimal release parameters and investigate the influence of the selection of release parameters (release angle, speed, and spin rate) on variability and success rate by comparing the theoretical and actual combinations of release parameters. This study could establish the computational method that can accurately connect the release parameters and the result, thus optimal release parameters by considering the effect of air drag and lift forces, which influences are not little. By using this method, it was revealed that players with a higher release position, a lower release speed, smaller variability in the anteroposterior arrival positions of the ball, and a larger margin for error for the release speed had higher success rate for FT shots. On the other hand, for 3P shots, players with a larger margin for error for the combination of the release speed and angle had higher success rate. However, the variabilities in release speed and angle did not have significant correlations with the success rate but the mean anteroposterior and absolute mean mediolateral distance and variabilities of it. Thus, it can be said that selecting the release parameters that allow the greater margin for error was important for increasing the success rate while keeping the variability low. These results suggest that simply computing the mean value and variability in release parameters cannot assess if players selected optical release parameters for maximizing success rate. However, computing the size of margin for error at selected release parameters enable us to assess if the selected release parameters are optimal. It must also be noted that traditional minimum-speed angles [2] were slightly larger than the new minimum-speed angles proposed in this study. Since increasing the margin for error for release parameters are important, and selecting unnecessary large release parameters can negatively influence the success rate by increasing the variability, computing optimal release parameters correctly is crucial.

For FT shots, there was a tendency that players who selected the release angle with larger margin for error for the release speed had higher success rate. It must be noted that this accompanied lower release speed and higher release height, which are assumed to have played a role in minimizing the variability in release speed as significant correlation between the release speed and SD of it was found in this study and reported by a previous study [1]. Thus, for FT shots, minimizing the variability in release speed by releasing the ball at higher position contributed to the higher success rate as well as having greater margin for error for release speed. As for the selection of release angle, no significant relation was observed to the success rate (Table 1). It is speculated that this was because the variability of release angles (2.0°) were relatively small compared to margin for error for release angle (12.7°) while for release speed, the variability was 0.12 m/s and the margin for error was 0.14 m/s. However, selecting release angle that is not unnecessarily high should be taken into consideration to minimize the variability in release angles, and minimizing the release speed as suggested as the idea of minimum-speed angle [2]. Using our new method of computing minimum-speed angle, the optimal release angle (46.9 ± 0.9°) was even smaller than the conventional method (47.7 ± 1.2°). Understanding the relationship between release parameters and the resultant trajectory, or the results of the shots appropriately will lead preventing misleading coaching to players to change release parameters.

For shots from a larger distance such as 3P in this study, it is difficult to maintain a low variability in the release speed since the amplitude of the necessary force is higher. However, in this study, variability in release parameters did not vary between FT and 3P (0.08 m/s and 1.3°). What influenced the success rate among the parameters related to anteroposterior direction was the mean arrival position (Table 3). These results suggest that though variability was kept low, tuning or grading the release parameters at the right magnitude was difficult for players, especially in longer distance shots. Thus, by selecting the release parameters that maximize the margin for error for both the release speed and the release angle resulted in higher success rate. If release angle had been simply increased in addition to the increased release speed in 3P from FT, it would have negatively affected the variability. Thus, the players with a higher success rate did not simply increase the release angle to increase the margin for error for the release speed, but selected the region that can maximize the margins for error for both release angle and speed, or near the minimum-speed angle.

The spin rate also had a significant effect on the successful combination of the release speed and angle. At the higher spin rate, the required speed at the selected release angle was reduced (Fig. 6). Also, the release speed that maximizes the margin for error for release angle and the minimum-speed angle were lower for the increased spin rate condition. It is assumed that by increasing the spin rate, the ball experienced greater lift force, which resulted in the trajectory with higher arch even when the ball was released at lower release speed. Thus, in addition to the reported positive influence of back spin at the interaction with the backboard and ring [5–8], our results added an insight that the trajectory is altered by the spin rate during the ball is in air.

References

1. Knudson, D.: Biomechanics of the basketball jump shot-six key teaching points. J. Phys. Educ. Recreat. Dance **64**, 67–73 (1993)
2. Brancazio, P.J.: Physics of basketball. Am. J. Phys. **49**, 356–365 (1981)
3. Miller, S.A., Bartlett, R.M.: The effects of increased shooting distance in the basketball jump shot. J. Sports Sci. **11**, 286–293 (1996)
4. Darling, W.G., Cooke, J.D.: Movement related EMGs become more variable during learning of fast accurate movements. J. Mot. Behav. **19**, 311–331 (1987)
5. Hamilton, G.R., Reinschmidt, C.: Optimal trajectory for the basketball free throw. J. Sports Sci. **15**, 491–504 (1997)
6. Silverberg, L., Tran, C., Adcock, K.: Numerical analysis of the basketball shot. J. Dyn. Syst. Measyrenebt Control **125**, 531–540 (2003)
7. Okubo, H., Hubbard, M.: Dynamics of the basketball shot with application to the free throw. J. Sports Sci. **24**(12), 1303–1314 (2006)
8. Tran, C.M., Silverberg, L.M.: Optimal release conditions for the free throw in men's basketball. J. Sports Sci. **26**(11), 1147–1155 (2008)
9. Okazaki, V.H.A., Rodacki, A.L.F.: Increased distance of shooting on basketball jump shot. J. Sport Sci. Med. **11**, 231–237 (2012)
10. Inaba, Y., Hakamada, N., Murata, M.: Influence of selection of release angle and speed on success rates of jump shots in basketball. In: Proceedings of the 5th International Congress on Sport Sciences Research and Technology Support – icSPORTS, pp. 48–55 (2017)
11. Yasuda, K., Tsuboi, K., Tanaka, K., Miyazaki, T.: Estimation of aerodynamic coefficients for a ball by using characteristics of trajectory. Trans. JSME **80**(814), 1–10 (2014)

Laboratory and Exercise Fitness Control in Young Soccer Players

Anna Zakharova, Kamiliia Mekhdieva[(⊠)], and Anastasia Berdnikova

Institute of Physical Education, Sport and Youth Policy,
Ural Federal University named after the first President of Russia B.N. Yeltsin,
620000 19 Mira Street, Yekaterinburg, Russia
sport_tsp@mail.ru, kamilia_m@mail.ru,
anastasia_berdnikova@mail.ru

Abstract. Athletes in prepubescent require a specialized approach to training process and its control, taking into consideration a broad range of physiological and training aspects in adolescents. The objective of the study was to evaluate fitness level of young soccer players and the search for interrelations between parameters of laboratory and field tests with the physiologic measurements during match play. The proposed paper provides coaches, sports scientists and physicians with important information on sufficient fitness control based on accessible and reliable tests. Twenty six healthy male soccer players born in 2004 aged 12–13 underwent the following laboratory testing: cycling stress-test with gas-exchange measurements, Wingate cycling test, performance analysis for vertical jumps and blood lactate measurements. Field tests included maximal interval running field test and jumping tests, as well as soccer game analysis with heart rate monitoring. Obtained data described overall parameters of young soccer players aged 12–13 from laboratory, field tests and game analysis with further comprehensive detailed interpretation. Significant interrelations between indicators of fitness condition, obtained from laboratory and field tests were found. For successful training management in young soccer players, laboratory and field tests should be widely used.

Keywords: Young soccer players · Training and testing · Field and laboratory tests

1 Introduction

Soccer has established itself as a popular worldwide, though demanding kind of sport. It is crucially important to consider such factors as:

- strength, power and agility, as they are valuable predictors of success in team sports and soccer in particular;
- anaerobic and aerobic abilities.

Technical and tactical skills are undoubtedly considered as the most valuable aspects in training process by coaches in soccer. However, in most cases these qualities are based on stated above factors.

J. Cabri et al. (Eds.): icSPORTS 2016/2017, CCIS 975, pp. 176–191, 2019.
https://doi.org/10.1007/978-3-030-14526-2_12

Successful training of a soccer team is determined by the timeliness and quality of the periodic control. The challenge of training planning in team sports is lack of objective criteria of fitness level assessment. Commonly, fitness level control in soccer implies monitoring and evaluation of physical abilities and in any type of sport measurements are to:

- correspond to the competitive activity, i.e. be specific;
- match the athletes' age and sport achievements as well as period of training;
- provide with informative and reliable data that appraise the athlete's current functional state, define strengths and weaknesses.

The appropriate control should consider specifics of soccer game – multiple-factor game activity. It is especially important in adolescent sports, when it is hard to forecast sport results, but at the same time it is required to prevent overreaching and over-training during intense training and game schedule. On the other hand, coaches and athletes themselves should avoid overestimation of abilities of young organism and expect too much at this age.

The key point is that due to prepubescent age characterized by intensive growth of an organism, external manifestations of lowered fitness level and sports results may be observed. However, the signs and potentials of successful athlete can be already found with the use of a wide range of laboratory tests.

In modern sport practice regular comprehensive control of the functional state of young soccer players makes sense. It is associated with the early age beginning of sport training in soccer, increase of training load at the initial stage of training, and moreover, with the high intensity in competition and its athletic character in the adult soccer. Hence, fitness control of young athletes should be mainly focused on objective assessment of internal factors of physical conditioning.

Notably, one of the issues we've faced nowadays is poor children's cardiovascular system development [30]. The reason is probably easy social, transport and living conditions in comparison with those of latter half of the twentieth century.

Thus in boyhood days it is extremely important to lay the foundation for specific physical fitness level and continuously monitor it to meet the requirements to the robust athlete in future soccer career.

It is commonly assumed that data obtained during the competition are the most reliable indicators of athletes' fitness level. Much information can be received from numerous portative sport devices, but heart rate belts and monitors are not permitted during official soccer matches [14, 26].

Modern functional diagnostics, computer technologies and digital devices in sports allow investigating various athletes' indicators which are important in sports activities. The only stumbling block is the set of methods and devices to be used. It is essential, that they must be limited in number, although provide with comprehensive information about physical competence. For research in a sport team it is required to choose the quickest testing procedure possible.

The purpose of this study was to describe and evaluate parameters of laboratory and field tests of young soccer players aged 12–13 years and define the most appropriate and indicative methods for athletes' fitness level assessment.

The correct choice of methods and procedures among the existing variety of those in modern sports practice could give coaches and sports scientists better understanding and working knowledge, in this way promoting sufficient training planning.

2 Organization and Methods

Twenty six healthy male soccer players born in 2004 currently aged 12–13 (height – 161.5 ± 7.32 cm, body mass – 49.5 ± 6.71 kg) were recruited for the study. The participants of the study had more than 5 years of sport experience in soccer. All subjects were free of cardiovascular or any other chronic disease. The investigation conforms to the principles of the Declaration of Helsinki of the World Medical Association. Athletes involved in the study had been provided with comprehensive information on the procedures, methods, benefits and possible risks before their parents' written consent was obtained and their permission was given. The study was approved by the Ural Federal University Ethics Committee.

2.1 Anthropometric Measurements

Weight and body composition were measured with the use of the MC-980MA Plus Multi Frequency Segmental Body Composition Monitor (TANITA, Japan) based on the advanced Bioelectric Impedance Analysis (BIA) technology. The following parameters were registered: body mass (kg), body mass index (BMI), muscle mass (kg; %), fat mass (kg; %), fat free mass (kg), bone mass (kg), intracellular and extracellular water (%), metabolic rate (kcal) and body mass balance.

2.2 Laboratory Exercise Testing

All laboratory tests were conducted in the research laboratory "Sports and health technologies" of the Institute of Physical education, sports and youth policy, UrFU. Laboratory exercise testing included maximal ramp cycling test with gas-exchange evaluation, cycling Wingate test and blood lactate measurements.

Maximal Ramp Cycling Test. Exercise testing was performed with the use of a bicycle ergometer ERG 911S (Schiller AG, Switzerland) and a desktop metabolic monitor Fitmate PRO (COSMED, Italy). Maximal ramp protocol was applied in accordance with ACC/AHA 2002 guideline update for exercise testing (2006) [1]. The test started from the load of 0 W during warm-up stage (1 min) with further load increase (40 W per minute). Athletes were recommended to keep the cadence about 80 rpm. The test was considered to have been performed at a maximal level of effort in case of: (1) the inability of the subject to maintain the expected cadence (80 rpm) despite verbal inciting; (2) refusal to continue the test due to subjective exhaustion of the muscles; (3) the appearance of absolute medical indicators. Maximal cycling test is widely used by sports physicians and practitioners in assessment of physical fitness and aerobic capacity. This type of protocol is quite informative, relatively safe and easily reproducible.

The following parameters were recorded starting with the first warm-up stage (1 min) and continuously during exercise testing: oxygen consumption (VO_2, ml kg^{-1} min^{-1}), heart rate (HR, bpm), stated exercise load (P,W), volume of ventilation (Ve, 1 min^{-1}), and respiration rate (Rf, 1 min^{-1}). The current values of all measured parameters were demonstrated on the metabolic analyzer screen and saved in the device memory for ongoing analysis.

Systolic blood pressure (SBP, mm Hg) and diastolic blood pressure (DBP, mmHg) were registered with the use of integrated blood pressure monitor (Schiller AG, Switzerland) after each second minute of the test. Immediate post-exercise measurements of HR, SBP and DBP during 5 min of recovery period were recorded. SBP and DBP values were manually fixed into metabolograph memory.

Gas-exchange measurements during stress test enabled us to obtain important information on athletes' aerobic capacity [28] and accurate values of metabolic changes under stress conditions. VO_{2max} – the maximal value of oxygen consumption during the test, anaerobic threshold (AT) and its relation to VO_{2max} (%) were determined through the stress-test. These indices characterize athletes' aerobic abilities and efficiency of oxygen utilization by working muscles.

A combination of the obtained physiologic characteristics during stress test with their further analysis provided with comprehensive information on integral response of respiratory apparatus, muscles and cardiovascular system to exercise load. In other words, it allowed estimating not only oxygen uptake, transport and utilization, but also efficiency of respiration at a maximal level of effort (Ve_{max}, 1 min^{-1} – maximal volume of ventilation per minute; Rf_{max}, 1 min^{-1} – maximal respiration rate; V_{max} – maximal volume of one inspiration) and muscle strength of athletes (P-VO_{2max} – the power reached at VO_{2max}). These indicators are considered as maximal individual for this particular type of test.

We also considered P_{170}, W – cycling power at a heart rate 170 beats per min, as a physical working capacity indicator similar to PWC_{170}-Cycle-test, the primary purpose of the which [6] is to predict the power output at a projected heart rate of 170 beats per minute (bpm). For example, one athlete attaines 180 W at the HR = 170 bpm while the other has only 150 W. The standard assumption is that the former is more physically fit than the latter.

Cycling Wingate Test. Cycling Wingate test was conducted with the use of the ergometer BIKE MED (TechnoGym, Italy) and Cardio Memory software V 1.0 SP3. Anaerobic power measures were obtained using leg cycling Wingate anaerobic test, and included peak power (PP, W), relative PP (W kg^{-1}), power at 15 (P_{15}, W) and 30 s (P_{30}, W), average power (AP_{30}) and their relative values (P_{15}, W kg^{-1}, P_{30}, W kg^{-1}, AP_{30}, W kg^{-1}).

Lactate Measurements. Blood lactate concentration (La, mmol l^{-1}) during performance testing of athletes was measured with the use of the portable device Vario Photometer DP 300 (Diaglobal, Germany) on microsamples of capillary blood from the fingertip. Post-exercise measurements of lactate were performed immediately after interval field testing and twice during the match (after the first and the second halves). It is well-known that lactate is the end product of the metabolic process of glucose utilization (anaerobic glycolysis) [13]. Thus, both in terms of the soccer game, as well as the interval running field testing, the rate of lactate elevation was considered as a measure of anaerobic abilities and a response to physical exertion.

Performance Analysis for Vertical Jumps. Performance analysis for vertical jumps is widely used tests in power and sprint sports [21, 27]. There were many ways to obtain data on the aspects of jumps parameters [18, 21, 27], but nowadays dynamics force plates are the demandable instruments to describe fast sport movement quantitatively. Kistler (Switzerland) – the leader in the field of sport performance analysis – uses piezoelectric sensors to measure forces and moments for sports and performance analysis. The more sensitive the force plate is, the more precise and reliable data are obtained.

The objectives of this part of study were (1) to obtain descriptive data on maximal anaerobic power output of the lower extremities with a force platform from counter-movement jump (CMJ) and squat jump (SJ) performed by soccer players and (2) to define issues in muscle realization of jumping.

Studied soccer players made three CMJs jumps and three SJs and the highest jumps of each player were analyzed. Athletes were instructed to perform the jumps with the maximum effort. All data were collected using two Kistler Jump force plates (type 9269AA3) with 64-channel block for data processing 5695B. MARS Software was used. Two platforms were used to obtain data from left and right leg separately. We were interested in the jump height (cm), relative maximal force (F) (%BW), relative maximal power (P) (W), push off time (s) and impulse (Ns) created by both legs and each leg separately in CMJ and SJ to assess imbalance in lower extremities muscles.

2.3 Field Soccer Tests

Maximal running interval testing was carried out on a pitch in a circle (lap) marked by 4 cones (20 m × 20 m). Athletes performed High Intensity Interval Training (HIITraining) of 8 sets of 20-second interval (Tabata Protocol) with an "all-out" effort separated by 10 s of passive recovery [22]. GPS Garmin Forunner 310XT was used to measure the distance length covered in each of 8 intensive bout and monitor heart rate (HR) during the HIIT-test and HR recovery after it. For quick and easy data access and HR and distance information acquisition and processing the GPS navigator configurations were installed on the interval training (12 intervals × 20 s + 10 s for rest). The additional 4 intervals were used for processing an athlete recovery data. According to the classification of training and competitive physical activities the highest result shown in the first cycle of the test corresponds to the zone of anaerobic alactic power (Dmax, m; Vmax, km/h) and it is the indicator of speed abilities [23] or athlete's running speed [31]. The sum of the first three results (D1-3), which depends mainly upon the degree of the covered distances decrease, serves as the marker of ability to maintain high speed. The result obtained within all 8 cycles corresponds to the work in anaerobic glycolic zone and the sum of 8 distances (D1-8) characterizes special stamina and anaerobic glicolytic potential of athlete's working muscle groups [23, 30].

All players were informed of the rating of the perceived exertion rating (RPE) scale (CR-10) and familiarized with it a month before the start of the study. The CR-10 scale proposed by Foster [11, 12] was presented to each player 12 min after Maximal running interval testing. This was done to exclude the influence of emotional factor after the test.

Jumping Tests. To define the strengths and weaknesses in leg muscles in field conditions one may use the results of jumping tests. It is well known that different types of jumps (hops or bounds) are performed by different muscles groups with particular prime mover in the certain type of jumps. Thus, double legs bounding are performed essentially by quadriceps, while standing bounds – by hip flexors and gluteus. Long jump is a complex manifestation of coordination, power and sport technique competence.

Comparison of jumping test results in a group permits to define averages. Those athletes who are in the top list with leg muscle strength of prime mover of the testing jump while regular monitoring the results in the same jumps during long period allow to follow the personal dynamics in strength development.

The performance of 1–3 jumps provide with the information on muscle power, 5 jumps – on strength and 10 jumps tell about strength endurance of leg muscles.

In our research we use the following jumping tests: long jump, 5 horizontal double legs bounding, tenfold standing bounds and tenfold single leg bounds on the right and left leg [25].

2.4 Soccer Game Analysis with Heart Rate Monitoring

To estimate age features of competitive activity of young soccer players the heart rate monitoring with GPS Garmin Forerunner 310XT (Garmin, USA) was used. HR was recorded every 5 s during each training session using HR monitor with individually coded HR transmitters to avoid interference. To measure the distance length covered during the game GPS navigation was used. Software Garmin Express and Garmin Connect helped us to determine the maximal velocity of young soccer-players, maximal and average HR, amount of time in different heart rate zones and others recovery speed.

The match (11 vs 11) was played on a regular size (105 × 68 m), synthetic-grass soccer pitch in two halves of 35 min (the official duration of the game for a given age of players), with 10-minute rest interval. During the game a ball of size 5 was used. To ensure that the game would restart immediately if the ball left the field of play, spare balls were kept all around the perimeter of the pitch. Six players were observed during the match.

The perceived exertion rating (RPE) scale (CR-10) was presented to each player 7 min after each half of the game.

2.5 Statistical Analysis

Statistical analysis was performed with the use of statistic software package "SPSS Statistics 17.0" (IBM). The descriptive analysis of the obtained data was applied to determine basic functional status of athletes. Normality of distribution was assessed by the Shapiro-Wilk test. Mean value (M) and standard deviation (SD) of the used parameters were calculated. Pearson correlations between the measured parameters were calculated to estimate the relations between results of laboratory, field and real-game measurements. The level of significance was set at $P < 0.05$.

3 Results and Discussions

The obtained data on anthropometric measurements of young soccer players (Table 1) [32] showed that generally athletes had age and gender appropriate body mass, height and most part of other parameters. High values of fat free mass (muscle mass) pointed at good physical status and beneficial training effect of soccer.

Table 1. Anthropometric and body composition analysis of young soccer players (12–13 years).

Parameters	M ± SD	(Min–max)
Height, cm	161.07 ± 7.64	149–176
Weight, kg	49.37 ± 6.41	36.8–61.7
CC, cm	73.65 ± 3.57	66–79
NC, cm	34.04 ± 2.13	30–39
MM, kg	38.85 ± 5.14	29.4–48.4
MM, %	78.59 ± 3	70.96–83.81
Fat, kg	8.48 ± 1.97	4.9–12.9
Fat, %	17.13 ± 3.15	11.7–25.1
BMI, kg/m^2	18.95 ± 1.54	16–21.5

CC – chest circumference; NC – neck circumference; MM – muscle mass.

Table 2 shows the results of laboratory cycling stress-test. On average, VO_{2max} in the studied group corresponded to high level in reference to age and gender norm in soccer for 12–13 years [10] and slightly lower one for age of 14.2 ± 0.5 years reported by Buchheit [4] VO_{2max} = 56.5 ± 0.9.

Average HR before the test, measured at rest sitting on cycle ergometer, was higher than sport norm. This result indicates the poor cardiovascular development that leads to

Table 2. Stress-test 4arameters of soccer players.

Parameters	M ± SD (min–max)	Athlete norm
VO_{2max}, ml kg^{-1} min^{-1}	54.34 ± 6.08 (45.8–66.6)	55
HR before the test, bpm	90.28 ± 10.59 (70–109)	70
HR$_{warming\ up}$, bpm	110.56 ± 8.3 (96–126)	85
HR $_{30w}$, bpm	113.22 ± 9.42 (95–129)	95
HR$_{max}$, bpm	182.89 ± 5.63 (172–192)	180–195
P$_{170}$,W	183.78 ± 35.14 (136–258)	–
P-VO$_{2max}$, W	222.67 ± 35.18 (152–294)	–
P-VO$_{2max}$/kg, W kg^{-1}	4.74 ± 0.46 (4.04–5.48)	>5
Ve$_{max}$, l min^{-1}	82.37 ± 16.97 (55.2–123.2)	>100
Rf$_{max}$, l min^{-1}	54.57 ± 12.98 (35.4–81.6)	45–52
V$_{max\ (Ve/Rf)}$, l	1.55 ± 0.45 (0.96–2.86)	>2
METS	15.56 ± 1.79 (13–19)	>15.5

HR – heart rate; P-VO$_{2max}$ – power reached at VO$_{2max}$; P-VO$_{2max}$/kg – relative maximum power at P-VO$_{2max}$; VO$_2$ – oxygen consumption; Ve$_{max}$ – maximal volume of ventilation; Rf$_{max}$ – maximal respiration rate; V$_{max}$ – maximal volume of one inspiration.

low aerobic abilities. At the same time HR_{max} was within athletic norm (Table 2), that means the balanced heart-muscle development of young soccer players. But this balance was reached thanks to good but not excellent power index (P-VO$_{2max}$/kg, W kg^{-1}). Meanwhile, most of the stress-test parameters varied within a certain range. This indicated considerable difference aerobic performance level and physical state of players of the same age.

As running speed and acceleration abilities are of great importance in soccer we reported opportunity to measure peak power in cycling Wingate test for testing of 11–12 years old [31]. No information about Wingate-test parameters at the age of 12 was found.

In the present study (Table 3) relative PP and AP were as high as the same indicators of 15–16 years old soccer players [15, 17] and higher than that of forwards [16] whereas all absolute values were lower. In comparison with 17 years old players with identical experience in soccer, the tested players showed lower values of PP, but the same values of AP [9]. This undoubtedly demonstrates the high level of leg muscles fitness for anaerobic work specific for soccer.

Table 3. Wingate-test parameters of soccer players.

Parameters	M ± SD (min–max)	Athletes' norm for 12–13 years
PP, W	517.21 ± 102.9 (371–698)	–
PP, w/kg	10.83 ± 1.24 (8.67–12.92)	≥ 11
P_{15}, W	421.71 ± 96.87 (292–628)	–
P_{15}, W/kg,	8.53 ± 1.12 (6.99–10.33)	–
P_{30}, W	337.71 ± 95.6 (226–497)	–
P_{30}, W/kg	6.78 ± 1.11 (5.06–9.15)	–
AP_{30}, W	415.29 ± 87.01 (314–607)	–
AP_{30}, W/kg	8.69 ± 0.96 (7.22–10.6)	≥ 9
Fatigue, %	41.29 ± 10.17 (25–62)	≤ 40
t_{pp}, s	5.64 ± 4.63 (2–17)	3–5

PP – peak power; AP – average power; t_{pp}, – time of PP attainment.

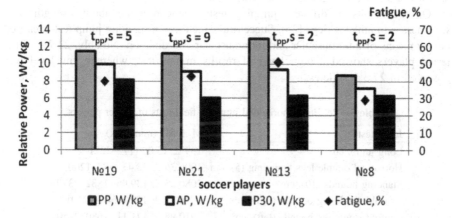

Fig. 1. Individual results of Wingate-test of soccer players.

Figure 1 demonstrates the individual results of Wingate-test. Player 19 demonstrated excellent power capabilities according to all Wingate parameters. Athlete 13 quickly reached peak power (PP = 12.92 W/kg, t_{pp} = 2 s) and showed high values of the average relative power but could not hold power throughout Wingate-test. Actually high value of fatigue linked with the insufficient development of power endurance of this player. The average values of all Wingate-test parameters were noted in athlete 21. His weak side was slow achievement of PP (t_{pp} = 9 s). Player 8 showed a lower level of anaerobic power and capabilities.

Table 4. Results of vertical jump tests of soccer players on a force platform

Parameters	Counter movement jump M ± SD (min–max)	Squat jump M ± SD (min–max)	P
Jump height from Take Off, cm	25.00 ± 3.11 (20.7–30.7)	28.4 ± 5.8 (20.2–37.2)	0.022
Relative maximal P, W/kg	40.75 ± 4.3 (34.94–48.74)	43.490 ± 5.202 (35.98–52.47)	0.021
Push off Time, s	0.272 ± 0.033 (0.212–0.318)	0.390 ± 0.069 (0.338–0.561)	0.00003
Impulse, Ns	110.98 ± 23.54 (74.99–150.8)	118.15 ± 25.322 (74.37–161.6)	0.017

Performance analysis for vertical jumps (Table 4) revealed a good preparedness tested players in the Counter Movement Jump (CMJ) in comparison with the average results of the European teenagers of 13 years (21.5 ± 6.6 cm) [24], young players (16.3 ± 1.26 years old) of the national team of Greece (elite group, 23.6 ± 3.5 cm) and players participating in the local championship of Greece (subelite group, 16.4 ± 1.32 years, 21.4 ± 4.5 cm), as well as in Squat jump (SJ) (23.4 ± 6.4 cm) [24]. Better values of jump height were demonstrated by adult soccer players (22.9 ± 2.8 years) of the third division of the Spanish Football League (CMJ – 40.73 ± 4.98 cm, SJ – 35.58 ± 5.2 cm) [29].

On the results of different jumping tests one can judge about strengths and weaknesses in athletes' legs [25]. Successful execution of the long jump test is carried out by means of intermuscular and intramuscular coordination. Notably, 22.7% of the tested players showed a high level of results in this test, whereas low level was observed in 27.3% athletes.

Table 5. Results of horizontal jumping field tests of soccer players.

Jump tests	M ± SD (min–max)
Long jump, cm	199 ± 15.06 (172–227)
Horizontal double legs bounding (5), cm	1006.36 ± 72.43 (885–1200)
Standing bounds (10), cm	2080.23 ± 139.06 (1882–2370)
Tenfold single leg bounds (right), cm	1916.73 ± 170 (1640–2210)
Tenfold single leg bounds (left), cm	1910.95 ± 171.11 (1680–2250)

In general, the tested players showed a high power level of leg muscles (Table 5). Excellent results of power of the knee joint extensors were registeredin 22.7% of the soccer players with the horizontal double legs bounding test (5 forward frog like jumps). Only 18.2% of athletes had low level of results in this test. The majority of young soccer players demonstrated correct execution of the horizontal double legs bounding technique, which requires certain muscular efforts and confirms the high level of strength preparedness at this age.

The performance of the 10 jumps requires strength endurance of the leg muscles [25]. Testing in standing bounds revealed that 27.3% of athletes had excellent strength endurance of the hip flexors and gluteus muscles. Typical mistakes of young players in this test were the lack of the qualitative first jump from two legs and a weak forward movement of the thigh which partially limited the phase of flight so necessary for the successful execution of the jump test.

A good and balanced development of ligaments and tendons of both feet, so important in soccer, was noted only in 22.7% of players. About 45.5% of young athletes demonstrated a balanced but insufficient level of preparedness in the tenfold single leg bounds test. The remaining 31.8% of tested players have a good development of ligaments and tendons but have a misbalance between the right and left legs. This is evidenced by the results of different tests: tenfold single leg bounds (SLB10-r, SLB10-l) (Table 5) and vertical jump tests on a force platform.

The results of interval running test are showed in Table 6 and Figs. 2 and 3.

ΔD (m) was calculated as the difference between the best interval and the interval with the minimum distance in the HIIT-test. This indicator ΔD (m) was adopted as a criterion of the ability to perform high-intensity running with minimal loss of productivity. The optimum value was assumed at $\Delta D \leq 30$ m.

Table 6. Results of interval running test of soccer players.

Parameters	M ± SD	Max
D_{max} per interval, m	114.45 ± 7.03	132
ΣD, m	746.82 ± 57.64	831
ΔD, m	31.82 ± 9.36	45
HR_{max}, bpm	189.36 ± 7.51	202
HR_{mean}, bpm	161.91 ± 6.22	171
V_{max}, km/h	20.6 ± 1.27	23.76
V_{mean}, km/h	16.8 ± 1.3	18.7
V_{min}, km/h	14.87 ± 1.69	17.1
ΔV, km/h	5.73 ± 1.19	8.1
La, mmol l^{-1}	7.89 ± 3.1	15.6
RPE	7 ± 1.41	9

D_{max} – distance covered in the best interval; ΣD – total distance for the test; ΔD – individual RPE – rate of the perceived exertion; La – capillary lactate concentration; V – velocity; ΔV – drop of the velocity during the test (between individual V_{max} and V_{min})

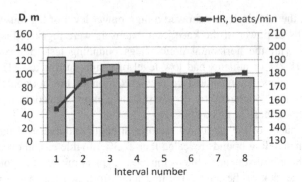

Fig. 2. The desirable excellent conditioning bar chat of young soccer players [32].

The desirable excellent conditioning bar chat of young football players is shown in Fig. 2.

The results of running interval test detected the physical fitness of every subject. The comparison and ranking of the first (best) distance results of all athletes reveal the winner in speed, while champion in 8 distances amount shows the desirable level of specific endurance (Fig. 3).

Many researchers have repeatedly performed the subsequent detailed analysis of external and internal load indicators, as well as technical and tactical preparedness of athletes during the played soccer matches [2, 7, 8, 19, 20]. The value of data obtained during the game cannot be overestimated. A variety of match analysis methods and tools allows not only to characterize one or several sides of a player's preparedness, but also to compare the obtained data with the results of the other tests. It is provided by short, but not less informative tests that do not require sophisticated equipment and huge energy costs for players (as during the game).

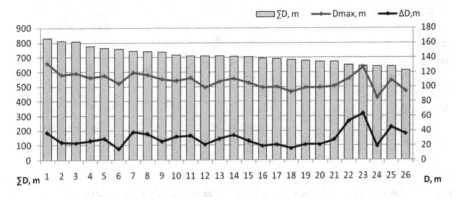

Fig. 3. Young soccer players (n = 26) individual results of interval running test.

During the whole game players (n = 12) covered 8500 ± 460 m (7930–8910 m), of which 4000 ± 550 m (3190–4560 m) were performed in the first half of the game and 4500 ± 500 (3910–5210 m) in the second half. The studied group of players showed a high level of the total distance covered per game in comparison with the data of other researchers in accordance with the age and gender norms in soccer (Barbero-Álvarez, 2013: age – 14.3 ± 1.3 years, total distance – 7145 ± 685 m; Buchheit [5]: age – U13, total distance – 6549 ± 597 m, age – U14, total distance – 7383 ± 640 m; Buchheit [4]: age – 14.2 ± 0.5, total distance – 5372 ± 125 m) [3–5].

The average and peak HR during the match were 160.5 ± 6.06 bpm (154–170 bpm) and 194.83 ± 6.94 bpm (range 188–206). The values of HR_{max} and HR_{mean} during the game were authentically lower than in Barbero-Álvarez study (2013) (HR_{max} – 205.7 ± 5.4 bpm, HR_{mean} – 179.7 ± 6.8 bpm) [3].

Lactate values after the first and second half of the game were 5.48 ± 2.28 mmol l^{-1} (2.87–9.25 mmol l^{-1}) and 3.71 ± 1.81 mmol l^{-1} (2.44–6.91 mmol l^{-1}) respectively. RPE response of players showed values of 4.17 ± 0.41 (4–5) and 5.5 ± 0.55 (5–6) after the first and second half of the game respectively.

During the match the players showed an average speed of 10.4 ± 1.61 km/h (7.6–11.54 km/h). The peak game speed was 20.4 km/h and it was lower than average values reported by Buchheit [5] about the players of the same age (age – U13, peak game speed – 22.3 ± 1.4; age – U14, peak game speed – 24.4 ± 1.8).

Taking into account the results of laboratory tests and field tests discussed above it can be assumed that low values of maximum speed during the game are associated with the game tactics but not with low fitness level of young players.

Data obtained from correlative analysis showed that there were strong interrelations between the parameters of physical fitness of young soccer players obtained from different tests.

In particular, we found significant correlations between PP and P-VO_{2max} (r = .805, P < 0.01), PP and P_{170} (r = .630, P < 0.05), AP and P-VO_{2max} (r = .822, P < 0.01), AP and P_{170} (r = .626, P < 0.05), AP and VO_{2max} (r = .566, P < 0.05).

Above-mentioned proves the interrelation between athletes' maximal power and strength manifestation in VO_{2max} protocol, or strange as it may seem between anaerobic power (PP, AP) and aerobic capacities in athletes. In other words, muscle strength abilities provide athletes with advantage in endurance, as shown in better physical characteristics during aerobic laboratory and field tests, as well as lower exertion during the game.

Moreover, close interrelations between parameters of Wingate test, vertical jumps performance analysis and field jumping tests were revealed. We found significant correlations between relative maximal P CMJ both legs and Wingate test indices: PP (r = .750, P < 0.05), PP/kg (r = .669, P < 0.05), AP (r = .772, P < 0.01), AP/kg (r = .711, P < 0.05), as well as between relative maximal P CMJ both legs with long jump (r = .809, P < 0.01), horizontal double legs bounding (r = .651, P < 0.05) and standing bounds (r = .732, P < 0.05). Jump height from take off correlated well with long jump (r = .651, P < 0.05), relative maximal F, % BW right leg correlated with horizontal double legs bounding (r = .698, P < 0.05).

In addition to stated above, we found strong correlations between the results of laboratory and field tests and measurements obtained during the soccer game. Our results showed that RPE during the game correlated with VO_{2max} ($r = -.622$, $P < 0.05$), La concentration after the 1st half well correlated with the following indices: PP ($r = .923$, $P < 0.01$), relative PP ($r = .934$, $P < 0.01$), AP ($r = .884$, $P < 0.05$), relative AP ($r = .841$, $P < 0.05$), D_{max} ($r = .859$, $P < 0.01$).

Concentration of La after the 2nd half correlated with $P\text{-}VO_{2max}$ ($r = -.946$, $P < 0.01$) and P_{170} ($r = -.898$, $P < 0.01$).

HR at 150 W during stress test correlated with the following indices of Wingate test: PP ($r = -.518$, $P < 0.05$), AP ($r = -.628$, $P < 0.01$), AP/kg ($r = -.640$, $P < 0.01$), HR_{max} at interval running field test ($r = .564$, $P < 0.05$) and La concentration after the 2nd half ($r = -.967$, $P < 0.01$); HR_{max} during interval running field test correlated well with HR_{mean} during the game ($r = .816$, $P < 0.05$).

Furthermore, we found the following relationship of external load indicators between HIIT-test and measurements obtained during the soccer game: distance covered in the first half of the game correlated with the total distance in HIIT-test (ΣD) ($r = .628$, $P < 0.05$) and D_{max} ($r = .629$, $P < 0.05$); distance covered in the second half of the game correlated with ΣD ($r = -.889$, $P < 0.05$), D_{max} ($r = -.746$, $P < 0.05$), D_{min} (minimum distance covered per interval) ($r = -.929$, $P < 0.05$).

The internal load indicators of the same tests also showed a good correlation. RPE after the 2nd half correlated with RPE of HIIT-test ($r = .71$, $P < 0.05$); HR_{max} during HIIT-test correlated well with HR_{mean} during the game ($r = .82$, $P < 0.05$) and HR_{max} during the game ($r = .63$, $P < 0.05$).

Figure 4 demonstrates the relation between the rate of the perceived exertion during the game and maximum oxygen consumption. One can see that the higher VO_{2max} was the lower rate of exertion athletes had after the game. Thus better abilities of oxygen consumption, transport and utilization in young soccer players provide them with better physical load tolerance during the game.

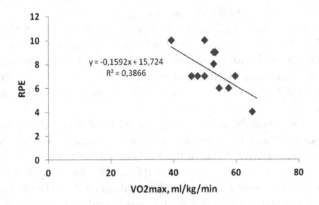

Fig. 4. Graph, describing relations between the rate of the perceived exertion (RPE) after the game and maximum oxygen consumption (VO_{2max}) [32].

4   Conclusions

1. Comprehensive fitness testing of soccer players aged 12–13 in laboratory and on the pitch revealed better-than-average physical condition. The fitness indicators of the young athletes in tested team corresponded to the general patterns of athletes' development of age mates in soccer. High fitness level of young players is a good basis for the further harmonious development that will provide the best conditions for manifestation of technical and tactical skills. Although, the limiting factor of exercise performance in tested soccer players is insufficient cardiovascular development.

2. Soccer players aged 12–13 demonstrated the following Wingate cycling test parameters: PP – 10.83 ± 1.24 W kg^{-1}, AP$_{30}$ – 8.69 ± 0.96 Wkg^{-1}, fatigue – $41.29 \pm 10.17\%$. Performance analysis for vertical jumps revealed high level of power of athletes. Soccer game analysis showed that adolescent soccer players covered the average distance of 8500 ± 460 m during 2×30 min game and demonstrated high physiologic response during the game: HR$_{max}$ – 194.83 ± 6.94 bpm, HR$_{mean}$ – 160.5 ± 6.06 bpm; La after the 1st half – 5.48 ± 2.28 mmol l^{-1}, La after the 2nd half – 3.71 ± 1.81 mmol l^{-1}.

3. For further professional career in soccer it is required to thoroughly monitor aerobic capacities of adolescent athletes and higher level of power abilities. VO$_{2max}$ not less than 55 ml kg^{-1} min^{-1} is a reliable predictor of success in team sport along with higher level of power which may be easily determined by means of Wingate test, force plate test and field jumping tests.

Acknowledgements. The work was supported by Act 211 Government of the Russian Federation, contract # 02.A03.21.0006.

References

1. ACC/AHA 2002 guideline update for exercise testing: summary article: a report of the American College of Cardiology/American Heart Association Task Force on practice guidelines. J. Am. Coll. Cardiol. **48**, 1731 (2006)
2. Aquino, R.L., et al.: Biochemical, physical and tactical analysis of a simulated game in young soccer players. J. Sports Med. Phys. Fitness **56**, 1554–1561 (2016)
3. Barbero-Álvarez, J.C., Pedro, R.E., Nakamura, F.Y.: Validity of a repeated-sprint ability test in young soccer players. Sci. Sports **28**(5), 127–131 (2013)
4. Buchheit, M., Delhomel, G., Ahmaidi, S.: Time-motion analysis of elite young French soccer players. Coach. Sport Sci. J. **3**, 21 (2008)
5. Buchheit, M., Mendez-Villanueva, A., Simpson, B.M., Bourdon, P.C.: Match running performance and fitness in youth soccer. Int. J. Sports Med. **31**, 818–825 (2010)
6. Cambell, P., et al.: Prediction of physical activity and physical work capacity (PWC 170) in young adulthood from childhood and adolescence with consideration of parental measures. Am. J. Hum. Biol. **13**, 190–196 (2001)
7. Castagna, C., D'ottavio, S., Abt, G.: Activity profile of young soccer players during actual match play. J. Strength Cond. Res. **17**, 775–780 (2003)

8. Castagna, C., Impellizzeri, F., Cecchini, E., Rampinini, E., Alvarez, J.C.B.: Effects of intermittent-endurance fitness on match performance in young male soccer players. J. Strength Cond. Res. **23**, 1954–1959 (2009)

9. Chtourou, H., Hammouda, O., Souissi, H., Chamari, K., Chaouachi, A., Souissi, N.: Diurnal variations in physical performances related to football in young soccer players. Asian J. Sport. Med. **3**(3), 139–144 (2012)

10. Cunha, G., Lorenzi, T., Sapata, K., Lopes, A.L., Gaya, A.C., Oliveira, Á.: Effect of biological maturation on maximal oxygen uptake and ventilatory thresholds in soccer players: an allometric approach. J. Sports Sci. **29**, 1029–1039 (2011)

11. Foster, C., Hector, L.L., Welsh, R., SchrageR, M., Green, M.A., Snyder, A.C.: Effects of specific versus cross-training on running performance. Eur. J. Appl. Physiol. **70**, 367–372 (1995)

12. Foster, C., et al.: A new approach to monitoring exercise testing. J. Strength Cond. Res. **15**, 109–115 (2001)

13. Goodwinn, M.L., et al.: Blood lactate measurements and analysis during exercise: a guide for clinicians. J. Diab. Sci. Technol. **1**, 558–569 (2007)

14. Impellizzeri, F.M.: Use of RPE-based training load in soccer. Med. Sci. Sports Exerc. **36**, 1042–1047 (2004)

15. Jastrzębski, Z., Barnat, W., Konieczna, A., Rompa, P., Radzimiński, Ł.: Changes of physical capacity and soccer-related skills in young soccer players within a one-year training period. Balt. J. Health Phys. Act. **3**(4), 248–261 (2011)

16. Joo, C.H., Seo, D.I.: Analysis of physical fitness and technical skills of youth soccer players according to playing position. J. Exerc. Rehabil. **12**, 548–552 (2016)

17. Júnior, J.B.S., da Silva Carvalho, R.G., Ferreira, J.C., da Silva, N.W.P., Szmuchrowski, L. A.: Correlação entre os índices do teste de corrida com o teste de Wingate. Arquivos em Movimento **4**(1), 12–22 (2010)

18. Lara, A., Abián, J., Alegre, L.M., Jiménez, L., Aguado, X.: Jump tests on a force platform for applicants to a sports science degree. J. Hum. Mov. Stud. **50**(2), 133–147 (2006)

19. Krustrup, P., Mohr, M., Ellingsgaard, H.E.L.G.A., Bangsbo, J.: Physical demands during an elite female soccer game: importance of training status. Med. Sci. Sports Exerc. **37**, 1242 (2005)

20. Mohr, M., Krustrup, P., Bangsbo, J.: Match performance of high-standard soccer players with special reference to development of fatigue. J. Sports Sci. **21**, 519–528 (2003)

21. Ntai, A., Zahou, F., Paradisis, G., Smirniotou, A., Tsolakis, C.: Anthropometric parameters and leg power performance in fencing. Age, sex and discipline related differences. Sci. Sports **32**(3), 135–143 (2017)

22. Tabata, I., et al.: Effects of moderate-intensity endurance and high-intensity intermittent training on anaerobic capacity and VO_{2max}. Med. Sci. Sports Exerc. **28**, 1327–1330 (1996)

23. Tarbeeva, N.: Method of Tabata interval training as a way of speed strength endurance control in cross country skiing. J. Uchenye zapiski universiteta imeni P.F. Lesgafta **76**(6), 156–159 (2011)

24. Ortega, F.B., et al.: Physical fitness levels among European adolescents: the HELENA study. Br. J. Sports Med. **45**(1), 20–29 (2011)

25. Shishkina, A.V.: Special power preparation of the qualified skiers-racers. J. Uchenye zapiski universiteta imeni P.F. Lesgafta, **3**(25), 99–103 (2007)

26. The International Football Association Board: Laws of the Game. FIFA, Zurich (2016)

27. Van Hooren, B., Zolotarjova, J.: The difference between countermovement and squat jump performances: a review of underlying mechanisms with practical applications. J. Strength Cond. Res. **31**(7), 2011–2020 (2017)

28. Vilikus, Z.: Functional Diagnostics, pp. 12–15. College of Physical Education and Sport, Palestra (2012)

29. Yanci, J., Los Arcos, A., Mendiguchia, J., Brughelli, M.: Relationships between sprinting, agility, one-and two-leg vertical and horizontal jump in soccer players. Kineziologija **46**(2), 194–201 (2014)

30. Zakharova, A., Berdnikova, A., Tarbeeva, A., Matvienko, V.: High intensity interval testing for fitness control of young football players. J. Uchenye zapiski universiteta imeni P.F. Lesgafta **124**(6), 70–75 (2015)

31. Zakharova, A.V., Berdnikova, A.N.: Monitoring of power abilities in young football players. Hum. Sports Med. **16**(4), 64–74 (2016)

32. Zakharova A., Mekhdieva K., Berdnikova A.: Comprehensive fitness control in young soccer players - comparison of laboratory and field testing indicators. In: icSPORTS 2017: Proceedings of the 5th International Congress on Sport Sciences Research and Technology Support Support, pp. 25–32 (2017)

Effects of Specific Badminton Training on Aerobic and Anaerobic Capacity, Leg Strength Qualities and Agility Among College Players

Eng Hoe Wee[✉], Jiun Yang Low, Kai Quin Chan, and Hui Yin Ler

Tunku Abdul Rahman University College, Jalan Genting Kelang,
53300 Kuala Lumpur, Malaysia
{weeeh, chankq, lerhy}@tarc.edu.my,
sethlow_4869@hotmail.com

Abstract. Multi-shuttle training was very popular and specific for the badminton training session. The badminton multi-shuttle feeding form possessed the quality of High Intensity Intermittent Training (HIIT) which resulted in physiological adaptations and improvement in physical performance. However, its effectiveness has not been extensively examined in badminton. This study examined the effects of high intensity intermittent badminton multi-shuttle (HIIBMS) feeding training on aerobic and anaerobic capacity, leg strength qualities and agility. Eighteen university college badminton players (AGE = 20 ± 1 year, BW = 65.3 ± 11 kg; H = 173.0 ± 5.3 cm) were recruited into this study. The subjects were pre-tested on aerobic capacity, leg reactive strength, and agility parameters. Subsequently, they were randomly selected and assigned into 2 groups (control group [CG], experimental group [EG]). Both groups had similar badminton training while additional training of HIIBMS feeding training was given to the EG for the duration of 4 weeks. The two groups started equal as the pre-test for the 6 research variables revealed insignificant results. The post-test results were also insignificant for all the 6 variables. However, pre-test and post-test mean scores comparisons showed significant improvements in VO$_2$max, mean power, leg reactive strength and agility except peak power and jump height in EG. CG showed no improvement in all parameters. Further research with longer intervention duration should be conducted to solicit for more information.

Keywords: Badminton training · Leg strength qualities · Anaerobic capacity

1 Introduction

Badminton is the most watched sport at the Olympics Games having attracted more than a billion spectators since its debut in 1996. It has become faster with increasing shot frequency, thus its physical demand is manifold requiring a mixture of technical and tactical skills, physiological fitness as well as psychological strength (Phomsoupha and Laffaye 2015). Numerous research (Andersen et al. 2007; Ooi et al. 2009; Jeyaraman and Kalidasan 2012) has reported badminton as a high intensity intermittent

© Springer Nature Switzerland AG 2019
J. Cabri et al. (Eds.): icSPORTS 2016/2017, CCIS 975, pp. 192–203, 2019.
https://doi.org/10.1007/978-3-030-14526-2_13

sport. It involved high intensity short effort, rapid change of direction, powerful leg and arm movements from various body position. As such badminton requires both the aerobic and anaerobic system in the physical performance and recovery.

Due to its high intensity intermittent nature, high intensity interval training (HIIT) has been accepted for training in badminton. HIIT has gained popularity in badminton due to its potentially large effects on exercise capacity coupled with the requirement of training duration was short (Foster et al. 2015). The similarity of HIIT and badminton intermittent nature has been supported by ACSM (2016). ACSM has accepted HIIT to be effective in improving sport performance through repeated bouts of high intensity effort followed by varied recovery interval similar to the movements and nature of badminton. Further, numerous studies (Laursen et al. 2005; Burgomaster et al. 2006; Gibala and McGee 2008; Little et al. 2011; Ziemann et al. 2011; Gibala et al. 2012) has reported that a short-term HIIT ranging from two weeks to six weeks could result in beneficial adaptations. Those studies had reported that HIIT was able to induce adaptations which were able to improve carbohydrate metabolism, increase in lactate transport capacity, oxidative energy provision, and lactate metabolism as well as overall exercise capacity. Even though the impact of HIIT on neuromuscular adaptation had not been looked into extensively, recent studies began to emphasize on the acute neuromuscular response towards HIIT training (Buchheit and Laursen 2013).

Multi-shuttle training (MST) is a popular method with a specific approach towards badminton training session (Han et al. 2011), similar to HIIT being widely used in sports training (Ziemann et al. 2011; Fernandez-Fernandez et al. 2012). MST involved lots of shuttles fed randomly or with specific drills to the trainee. In addition, MST could solicit different types of training goals, including tactical, technical and physical (Han et al. 2011; Hamedinia et al. 2013). Apparently the literature on the effectiveness of MST is sparse. As such, this study examined the effects of high intensity intermittent multi-shuttle on aerobic and anaerobic capacity, reactive leg strength and agility among college badminton players.

2 Methods

2.1 Participants

A total of 18 male university college badminton players (age = 20 ± 1 year; weight = 65.3 ± 11 kg; height = 173.0 ± 5.3 cm) were identified and invited for this study. Previous similar studies used 12 to 31 subjects, thus based on those studies the sample size of this study was considered adequate (Walklate et al. 2009 [n = 12, CG = 6, EG = 6]; Ziemann et al. 2011 [n = 21: CG = 11, EG = 10]; Fernandez et al. Fernandez et al. 2012 [n = 32: CG = 9, EG1 = 11, EG2 = 12]; Abdullah 2014 [n = 16: EG = 8, CG = 8]). Prior to the commencement of this study, the Physical Activity Readiness Questionnaire (PAR-Q) was administered to rule out contraindications to participation. PAR-Q results showed that all the subjects were healthy and free of any chronic health conditions. The subjects also signed the consent form after the briefing on the methods, procedures, benefits and potential risk. This procedure conformed with the principles of the declaration of Helsinki of the World Medical Association. The University College Ethics Committee has granted approval to this study.

2.2   Research Design

The design of this study was pre-test-intervention-post-test. The subjects were randomly select and divided into 2 groups (control and experimental) after pre-tests on aerobic, anaerobic (mean and peak power), reactive strength and agility parameters. The selection of subjects into the 2 groups were based on the total Z-scores of the 6 tests and systematic counter balancing method was used to assigned them into the 2 groups. Fishbowl method was used to assign the 2 groups into Control Group (CG) and Experimental Group (EG). Both the CG and EG groups underwent normal badminton training routines for four weeks. EG had an additional High Intensity Intermittent Badminton Multi-shuttle training (Fig. 1) while CG has none.

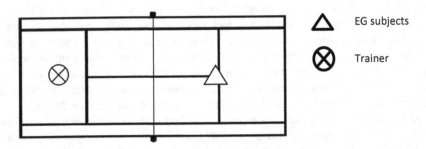

Fig. 1. Multi-shuttle training. Source: Wee et al. (2017). Proceedings from icSPORTS 2017: The 5th International Congress on Sport Sciences Research and Technology Support. Lisbon, Portugal: Science and Technology Publications.

2.3   Exercise Testing

The subjects of this study were subjected to the Bruce Protocol, Wingate Test, Countermovement Vertical Jump, Drop Jump and Illinois Agility Test. All tests were conducted in the laboratory and were based on the training schedule. In order to measure aerobic capacity, Treadmill (COSMED T200) and metabolic system (COSMED QUARK CPET) were used. Prior to the tests, all the subjects were required to warm up at a walking speed for 8–10 min. After the warming up session, the subjects started the test by running at an incline/gradient of 10% and a speed of 2.74 km/h. The incline and speed of the treadmill were increased every three minutes. The gradient was increased by 2% at every level. The subject ran to fatigue. Four conditions were monitored during the test to ensure subject achieved maximum capacity: 1. Plateau in oxygen uptake (<2 ml.kg/min or 3% with an increase in exercise intensity), 2. The respiratory ratio of 1.15 or above, 3. The final heart rate of within 12 bpm of the predicted age-related maximum, and 4. An RPE of 19 or 20 on the Borg Scale. Anaerobic capacity was measured using Braked Cycle Ergometer (883E Sprint Bike, Monark, Sweden). The test protocol involved all participants to start with a standardized 5-min warm-up cycling at 25 W. In the last seconds of the warm-up period, the subject increased their pedal rate to >100 rpm with no resistance. After a rest for 5-min, the test began from a stationary starting position with the participant seated at the right pedal at approximately 45 degrees. A resistance pedalling equal to 0.075 kp per kg of body mass was applied at the onset of the Wingate Test (Ayalon et al. 1974). The subjects then attempted to maximize their pedalling rate for the next 30 s under the prescribed resistance. Mean power and peak power generated from Monark anaerobic Test Software (Version 3.3.0.0) were used as an indicator of anaerobic capacity and was expressed in W/kg.

Leg reactive strength was measured using force plate (Bertec FP4060-10-4000, $\alpha = 0.978$ [pilot]). Subjects were instructed to drop from a 30 cm plyometric box. The box was positioned directly behind a force plate. Initially, the force platform was set to zero without the participant on the platform. The participants were reminded to limit their ground contact time (GCT) between the drop from the box and the jump. To begin, participant stepped off the box and dropped onto the force plate landing with both feet and jump as high as possible. The jump height was calculated using the formula: Jump height = 9.81 * (flight time)2/8. The best of three trials with GCT under 250 ms was used for analysis. The height in mm was divided by the time on the ground in milliseconds to determine the reactive strength index. To determine muscular power, Countermovement Vertical Jump Test was used ($\alpha = 0.89$, Fah 2012). Calculation of jump height was similar to reactive strength. Illinois Agility Test was used to measure agility ($\alpha = 0.965$, Lim et al. 2012).

2.4 Multi-shuttle Training

For this study, the multi-shuttle feeding training program was conducted for 4 weeks. Each training session consisted of 3 sets of 10 repetitions workouts. In between each set, 1 min rest was given. Each repetition consisted of 15 s of high-intensity work followed by 30 s rest. In the 15-s workout, the experimental subjects hit 8 shuttles which were fed by the trainer. The shuttle feeding was standardized with the trainer serving the shuttles with a badminton racket. In order to control the frequency of shuttle feeding, the metronome in Garmin Fenix 3 watch was used. The trainer kept feeding the shuttles to maintain high intensity in accordance to the rhythm of the metronome. The experimental subjects heart rate responses were monitored by a heart rate monitor connected to Garmin Fenix 3. The heart rate was recorded at the end of each set (Fig. 2).

The heart rate (HR) of EG subjects were monitored by Garmin Fenix 3 to ensure high intensity training and high stress (HR ranging from 165 bpm to 185 bpm) in accordance with Ghosh (2008) recommendation. The HR responses of the EG subjects were illustrated in Fig. 2. The bar charts for 3 sets and 12 training sessions revealed that the HR responses were 80% and above of maximal heart rate (MHR). This HR response was in accordance to the suggestion by Gibala (2015). Gibala recommended that the targeted heart rate should be between 80–100% of MHR to stimulate related adaptations.

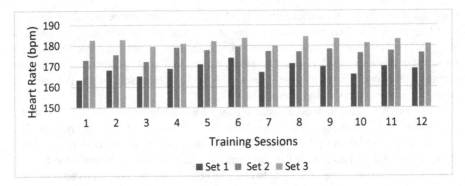

Fig. 2. Heart rate response in each training session across 12 sessions for 4 weeks as measured by Garmin Fenix 3. Source: Wee et al. 2017. Proceedings from icSPORTS 2017: The 5th International Congress on Sport Sciences Research and Technology Support. Lisbon, Portugal: Science and Technology Publications.

2.5   Statistical Analysis

Descriptive statistics for the research parameters such as means and standard deviations were used to report the basic data of the study. The descriptive statistics also discussed the background information of the subjects which included age, sports training background, and badminton experience. The test results were collected through VO2max Test, Wingate Bike Test, Drop Jump, Vertical Jump and Illinois Agility Test.

All the data was analysed using SPSS 23 for Windows software (IBM Corp, Armonk, NY, USA). The hypotheses of this study were tested using paired sample t-test and independent sample t-test. Paired sample t-test was used to compare the pre-test and post-test mean scores of the EG as well as the CG. Independent sample t-test was used to compare the pre-test mean scores of EG and CG as well as the post-test mean scores of both groups. The level of significance was set at $p < 0.05$.

3   Results

As shown in Table 1, descriptive analysis of the pre-test results showed both EG and CG were similar in all the six parameters. However, in the post-test, EG performed better than CG in VO2max, mean power and RSI, while CG performed better than EG in peak power, jump height and Illinois Agility test. The comparison of the pre-test and post-test mean scores of the two groups revealed that EG has the greatest improvement in VO2max and leg reactive strength respectively 10.08% (from 48.5 ml/kg/min to 53.4 ml/kg/min) and 41.53% (from 0.93 to 1.32) as compared to CG. While EG showed a slight improvement in mean power, vertical jump, and agility as compared to CG.

Table 1. Comparison of VO₂max, mean power, peak power, jump height, reactive leg strength and agility between the experimental group and control group. data are means (± SD) and percentage improvement. Source: Wee et al. 2017. Proceedings from icSPORTS 2017: The 5th International Congress on Sport Sciences Research and Technology Support. Lisbon, Portugal: Science and Technology Publications.

Variable	Experimental group			Control group		
	Pretest	Posttest	%of improvement	Pretest	Posttest	% of improvement
VO₂max (ml/kg/min)	48.5 ± 8.4	53.4 ± 6.7	10.08%	47.2 ± 12.00	46.9 ± 12.28	−0.73%
Mean power (W/kg)	7.80 ± 0.89	8.10 ± 0.69	3.74%	7.S6 ± 7.0	7.85 ± 0.79	2.38%
Peak power (W/kg)	10.61 ± 0.98	10.64 ± 0.94	0.24%	10.65 ± 0.86	10.74 ± 0.90	0.86%
Jump height (m)	0.39 ± 0.08	0.41 ± 0.07	5.76%	0.43 ± 0.09	0.44 ± 0.008	1.54%
Reactive strength (RSI)	0.93 ± 0.39	1.32 ± 0.42	41.53%	1.06 ± 0.14	1.11 ± 0.40	4.82%
Agility (s)	17.66 ± 0.76	17.09 ± 0.69	3.23%	17.56 ± 0.96	17.58 ± 0.94	−0.11%

When the pre-test mean scores of EG and CG (Table 2) were compared, the inferential statistics revealed that there were no significant differences in the pre-tests of all the six parameters of VO2max (0.263, p = 0.796), Mean Power (0.37, p = 0.716), Peak Power (−0.09, p = 0.93), Jump Height (−1.221, p = 0.24), Reactive Leg Strength (−0.677, p = 0.508) and Agility (0.259, p = 0.799). The results showed that EG and CG started equal before the intervention. Thus if post-test showed significant results, then the intervention program could be successful. Similar results were reported for post-test. The results in Table 3 revealed that all the 6 parameters measures were not significantly different when EG and CG were compared; VO2max (1.398, p = 0.181),

Table 2. A comparison of VO2max, mean power, peak power, jump height, reactive strength and agility pre test mean scores between experimental group and control group. Source: Wee et al. 2017. Proceedings from icSPORTS 2017: The 5th International Congress on Sport Sciences Research and Technology Support. Lisbon, Portugal: Science and Technology Publications.

Variable	Group	Mean	df	SD	t-value	Sig.
VO₂max	EG	48.5 ± 8.4	16	8.4	0.263	0.796
	CG	47.22 ± 12.0		12.0		
Mean power	EG	7.80 ± 0.89	16	0.89	0.37	0.716
	CG	7.66 ± 0.70		0.7		
Peak power	EG	10.61 ± 0.98	16	0.98	−0.09	0.93
	CG	10.65 ± 0.86		0.86		
Jump height	EG	0.39 ± 0.08	16	0.08	−1.221	0.24
	CG	0.43 ± 0.09		0.09		
RSI	EG	0.93 ± 0.39	16	0.39	−0.677	0.508
	CG	1.06 ± 0.14		0.14		
Illinois agility test	EG	17.66 ± 0.76	16	0.76	0.259	0.799
	CG	17.56 ± 0.96		0.96		

*The mean difference is significant at the .05 levels

Mean Power (0.713, p = 0.486), Peak Power (−0.242, p = 0.812), Jump Height (−0.899, p = 0.382), Reactive Leg Strength (1.057, p = 0.306) and Agility (−1.246, p = 0.231). However, when the pre-test and post-test performance were compared for both groups (Table 3), it was found that there were no significant differences in all the 6 parameters for CG but significant differences were found for EG in VO2max, Mean power, Reactive Strength and Agility.

Table 3. A comparison of VO2max, mean power, peak power, jump height, reactive strength and agility between pre-test and post-test mean scores in experimental group and control group. Source: Wee et al. 2017. Proceedings from icSPORTS 2017: The 5th International Congress on Sport Sciences Research and Technology Support. Lisbon, Portugal: Science and Technology Publications.

Variable	Group	Pre-test	Post-test	df	t-value	Sig.
VO2max	EG	48.5 ± 8.4	53.4 ± 6.7	8	−4.73	0.001*
	CG	47.2 ± 12.00	46.9 ± 12.28	8	0.40	0.701
Mean power	EG	7.80 ± 0.89	8.10 ± 0.69	8	−2.41	0.042*
	CG	7.66 ± 7.0	7.85 ± 0.79	8	−1.93	0.089
Peak power	EG	10.61 ± 0.98	10.64 ± 0.94	8	−0.11	0.915
	CG	10.65 ± 0 86	10.74 ± 0.90	8	−0.45	0 663
Jump height	FG	0.39 ± 0.08	0.41 ± 0.07	8	−1.74	0.12
	CG	0.43 ± 0.09	0.44 ± 0.08	8	−0.63	0.545
Reactive strength (RSI)	EG	0.93 ± 0.39	1.32 ± 0.42	8	−5.15	0.001*
	CG	1.06 ± 0.14	1.11 ± 0.40	8	1.29	0.233
Agility	EG	17.66 ± 0.76	17.09 ± 0.69	8	6.79	0.000*
	CG	17.56 ± 0.96	17.58 ± 0.94	8	0.43	0.681

*The mean difference is significant at the .05 level

4   Discussions

The purpose of this study was to investigate the effects of high intensity intermittent multi-shuttle badminton training on aerobic and anaerobic capacity, leg reactive strength and agility.

The result of the post-test in this research showed no significant difference between EG and CG in all the 6 parameters (VO2max, mean power, peak power, jump height, reactive leg strength, agility). This has diminished the potential of HIIT in affecting large exercise capacity within a short duration, Even though EG has undergone a 4-week intervention (badminton multi-shuttle training), three 30 min sessions weekly, the result was not similar to that of Gillen and Gibala (2014). Gillen and Gibala (2014) reported that as little as three 10 min sessions weekly, with only 3 x 20 s high intensity, could affect both muscle oxidative capacity and several markers of cardio-metabolic health even though this investigation employed 10 x 3 x 15 s HIIT. Selier et al. (2013) has suggested that larger volume of training should be used. Individuals interested in enhancing outcomes (including competitive performance) should regularly do both a larger volume of training and higher intensity training.

4.1 Effect of High Intensity Intermittent Multi-shuttle Feeding Training on Aerobic Capacity

The results of this research showed a significant improvement in VO2max. The improvement was 10.08% (p = 0.001) in EG and 0.73% (p = 0.701) in CG. The significant improvement in EG's VO2max was similar to the finding of Sloth et al. (2013). Sloth et al.'s (2013) reported that the effects of a high-intensity interval training usually increased VO2max by 4.2–13.4%. Further, the increment of 4.9 ml/kg/min VO2max corresponded to Ziemann et al. (2011) finding that an improvement of 5.5 ml/kg/min VO2max with a similar work-rest ratio interval training (1:2 work-rest ratio) on similar population (active college-aged men). On the contrary, CG (−0.3 ml/kg/min) had a decrement in VO2max. CG only had 3 regular sessions of fewer than 2 h training volume of match play per week. In the context of the improved VO2max, it might be explained by increased oxygen availability due to central adaptations or as a result of peripheral adaptations. However, the central adaptations were less likely to happen through the present study's training protocol as the effects on cardiac function would need peak-load (high intensity) durations of at least 2 or 3 min (Buchheit and Laursen 2013) and training period of 8 weeks must be applied (Matsuo et al. 2014).

The MST feeding training consisted of change of direction (COD) elements where the athletes moved from one corner to another corner quickly during the 15 s work phase. The inclusion of COD into HIIT had been proven to place high stress on the athletes regardless of the duration of the work interval (10 s to 30 s) (Dellal et al. 2010) and this has helped improved VO2max of EG. In addition, Buchheit and Laursen (2013) highlighted that the peripheral as well as systemic cardiorespiratory system demand were higher during the COD type of HIIT, and this explained the significant improvement of VO2max in EG. The effects of COD elements during sport skill training on VO2max was reported by Karahan (2012).

4.2 Effect of High Intensity Intermittent Multi-shuttle Feeding Training on Aerobic Capacity

This study revealed significant improvement of 3.74% in the mean power of EG and insignificant improvement in CG (2.38%). In the case of peak power, both EG and CG showed insignificant improvement of 0.24% and 0.86% respectively. The percentage improvement of the mean power and peak power of this investigation was much less if the studies of Foster et al. (2015), and Ziemann et al. (2011) were compared. Ziemann et al. (2011) found 6-week HIIT program favourably influenced the aerobic and anaerobic performances of college subjects. On the contrary, the improvement in the anaerobic capacity through HIIT multi-shuttle feeding training in this study was consistent with Walklate et al.'s (2009) finding in which the badminton players showed improvement in anaerobic parameters after involving in a 4-weeks badminton agility sprint training. In supporting this result, Karahan (2012) reported an improvement of 10.7% in the mean power of a skill-based HIIT training. Further, this was confirmed by Laursen et al. (2005) who observed that 4 weeks of HIIT could helped increased the anaerobic capacity as evaluated through accumulated oxygen deficit.

4.3   Effect of High Intensity Intermittent Multi-shuttle Feeding Training on Reactive Leg Strength

Reactive strength is related to accelerated speed, change of direction speed, and even agility. It is similar to the movements of EG subjects moving from the middle of the court to the corner where the shuttle was placed and returned to the middle of the court again. This could explain the result of this study where the reactive strength index demonstrated a significant improvement of 41.53% in EG and insignificant improvement of 4.82% in CG.

However, the findings of this study showed insignificant improvement in jumping height (5.76%) for EG and CG (1.54%). In supporting this result, Vissing et al. (2008) emphasised that the improvement of agility related factor (leg strength) was relatively smaller in trained subjects who were familiarized with stretch-shortening cycle (SSC) exercise patterns. In this study, the EG subjects were trained badminton players.

The MST involved changes of direction (COD) movements. Numerous studies such as that of Gamble (2012) and Young, Dawson and Henry (2015), observed that COD was highly correlated to reactive strength, thus that explained the improvement in the reactive strength in EG. Conversely, Born et al. (2016) in examining the effects of multi-directional interval sprinting training on change of direction ability failed to support the result of this research.

4.4   Effect of High Intensity Intermittent Multi-shuttle Feeding Training on Leg Power

The findings of this study revealed insignificant improvement in leg power in EG (5.76%) and CG (1.54%). In supporting this finding, McBride, McCaulley and Cormie (2008), concur that power involved in longer stretch-shortening cycle (SSC) compare to reactive strength. Since the multi-shuttle training was analogous to plyometric training which involved high force application and brief ground contact time (Gamble 2012), the contribution of the slower SSC was less. Thus the transfer of the adaptation might be more specific towards reactive strength instead of leg power.

4.5   Effect of High Intensity Intermittent Multi-shuttle Feeding Training on Agility

This study reported significant improvement of 3.23% of agility in EG and insignificant agility result for the CG (decrement of 11%). Rathore (2016) explained that the significant result in EG, might be due to the fact that the court movements in the high intensity intermittent multi-shuttle feeding training were similar to plyometric training drills involving explosive stopping, starting, and changing direction movements. This could be supported by the fact that the phenomenon of the stretch-shortening cycle (SSC) was especially prevalent in an intermittent game like badminton. SSC actions exploited the myotatic reflex as well as the elastic qualities of tendons and muscle, and the resulting performance is independent of maximum strength in players.

The EG subjects played on one side of the court and they were fed with shuttles from the opposite side by a coach. The subjects would rush to the backline and returned the shuttle executing required stroke from the back line, moving back to the center of the court. As half-court was of smaller size, explosive movements such as jumping, turning, initiation of movement, lateral movements and agility were more important than maximum speed (Kusuma et al. 2015). In supporting this observation, Walklate et al. (2009) emphasized that the badminton specific repeated sprints conditioning intervention compromised a sequence of rehearsed movements covering the court and resulted in improvement of repeated sprint agility performance and anaerobic capacity. Further, Lim et al. (2012) reported that the movements during the multi-shuttle training which included the change of direction movements involved performing the correct movements, performing accelerations and decelerations toward the shuttlecock, and performing sharp changes of direction or backpedaling. Holmberg (2009) supported this finding stating that agility was an acquired motor skill that could be trained. He stressed that badminton players could improve agility through technical training, pattern running and reactive training. Potteiger et al. (1999) agreed that improvements in agility were a result of enhanced motor unit recruitment patterns. As a result of training, neural adaptations occurred in athletes. These adaptations consequently improved the coordination between CNS signal and proprioceptive feedback in athletes (Craig 2004). This finding was also supported by Salonikidis and Zafeiridis (2008) which reported that their research subjects who underwent the tennis-specific drills training improved their speed and quickness of movement. These observations has indicated that the sports specific training in racket games could contribute to the improvement in agility.

5 Conclusions

The purpose of this study was to investigate the effects of high intensity intermittent multi-shuttle badminton training on aerobic and anaerobic capacity, leg reactive strength and agility. The findings on the sample of college badminton players has suggested that there was no particular advantage for high intensity multi-shuttle training model except some improvement for few variables for EG.

6 Future Research Direction

The findings of this research might be limited by the four weeks duration of the experiment. Thus, a longer duration is suggested in future research. Further, it could be postulated that the differences in skill level among the college badminton players might affect the adaptive response towards the training. Therefore, it is suggested that for future research, the skill levels of badminton players should be taken into consideration.

References

ACSM: ACSM's Guidelines for Exercise Testing and Prescription, 9th edn. Lippincott Williams & Wilkins, Philadelphia (2016)

Abdullah, S.: Effect of high intensity interval circuit training on the development of specific endurance to some of essential skills in youth badminton players. J. Adv. Soc. Res. **4**(3), 77–85 (2014)

Andersen, L.L., Larsson, B., Overgaard, H., Aaggard, P.: Torque-velocity characteristics and contractile rate of force development in elite badminton players. Eur. J. Sport. Sci. **7**(3), 127–134 (2007)

Ayalon, A., Inbar, O., Bar-Or, O.: Relationships among measurements of explosive strength and anaerobic Power. International Series on Sport Sciences, pp. 572–577 (1974)

Born, D.P., Zinner, C., Duking, P., Sperlich, B.: Multi-directional sprint training improves change-of-direction speed and reactive agility in young highly trained soccer players. J. Sport. Sci. Med. **15**(2), 314–319 (2016)

Buchheit, M., Laursen, P.B.: High-intensity interval training, solutions to the programming puzzle: part ii: anaerobic energy, neuromuscular load and practical applications. Sport. Med. **43**(10), 927–954 (2013)

Burgomaster, K.A., Heigenhauser, G.J.F., Gibala, M.J.: Effect of short-term sprint interval training on human skeletal muscle carbohydrate metabolism during exercise and time-trial performance. J. Appl. Physiol. **100**(6), 2041–2047 (2006)

Craig, B.W.: What is the scientific basis of speed and agility? Strength Cond. J. **26**(3), 13–14 (2004)

Dellal, A., Keller, D., Carling, C., Chaouachi, A., Wong, D.P., Chamari, K.: Physiologic effects of directional changes in intermittent exercise in soccer players. J. Strength Cond. Res. **24** (12), 3216–3219 (2010)

Fah, P.W.: Effects of zig-zag training on the female volleyball player's leg power performance. Advanced Diploma in Sport and Exercise. Tunku Abdul Rahman College (2012)

Fernandez-Fernandez, J., Zimek, R., Wiewelhove, T., Ferrauti, A.: High-intensity interval training vs repeated-sprint training in tennis. J. Strength Cond. **26**(1), 53–62 (2012)

Foster, C., et al.: The effects of high intensity interval training vs steady state training on aerobic and anaerobic capacity. J. Sport. Sci. Med. **14**, 745–755 (2015)

Gamble, P.: Training for Sports Speed and Agility: An Evidence-Based Approach. Routledge, New York (2012)

Gibala, M.J., McGee, S.L.: Metabolic adaptations yo short-term high-intensity interval training: a little pain for a lot of gain? Exerc. Sport Sci. Rev. **36**(2), 58–63 (2008)

Gibala, M.J., Jonathan, P.L., MacDonald, M.J., Hawley, J.A.: Physiological adaptations to low-volume, high-intensity interval training in health and disease. J. Physiol. **590**(5), 1077–1084 (2012)

Ghosh, A.K.: Heart rate and blood lactate responses during execution of some specific strokes in badminton drills. Int. J. Appl. Sports Sci. **27**(2), 27–36 (2008)

Gibala, M.: Physiological adaptations to low-volume high-intensity interval training. Sports Sci. Exch. **28**(139), 1–6 (2015)

Gillen, J.B., Gibala, M.J.: Is high-intensity interval training a time-efficient exercise strategy to improve health and fitness? Appl. Physiol. Nutr. Metab. **39**, 409–412 (2014)

Hamedinia, M.R., Saburi, H., Moeinfard, M.R.: A survey on annual periodization of the iranian skillful male badminton coaches. Int. J. Sport Stud. **3**(9), 970–977 (2013)

Han, Y., Li, S., Wang, R.: An insight of the application of multi-shuttle training in badminton. The 4th sport science and recreational activity management thesis collection, pp. 75–80 (2011)

Holmberg, P.M.: Agility training for experienced athletes: a dynamical systems approach. Strength Cond. J. **31**(5), 73–78 (2009)

Jeyaraman, R., Kalidasan, R.: Prediction of playing ability in badminton from selected anthropometrical physical and physiological characteristics among inter collegiate players. Int. J. Adv. Innov. Res. **1**, 47–58 (2012)

Karahan, M.: The effect of skill-based maximal intensity interval training on aerobic and anaerobic performance of female futsal players. Biol. Sport **29**(3), 223–227 (2012)

Kusuma, D.W.Y., Raharjo, H.P., Taathadi, M.S.: Introducing a new agility test in badminton. Am. J. Sport. Sci. **3**(1), 18–28 (2015)

Laursen, P.B., Shing, C.M., Peake, J.M., Coombes, J.S., Jenkins, D.G.: Influence of high intensity interval training on adaptations in welltrained cyclists. J. Strength Cond. Res. **19**, 527–533 (2005)

Lim, J.H., Wee, E.H., Chan, K.Q., Ler, H.Y.: Effect of plyometric training on the agility of students enrolled in required college badminton programme. Int. J. Appl. Sport. Sci. **24**(1), 18–24 (2012)

Little, J.P., et al.: Low-volume high-intensity interval training reduces hyperglycemia and increases muscle mitochondrial capacity in patients with type 2 diabetes. J. Appl. Physiol. **111** (6), 1554–1560 (2011)

Matsuo, T., et al.: Effects of a low-volume aerobic-type interval exercise on VO2max and cardiac mass. Med. Sci. Sport. Exerc. **46**(1), 42–50 (2014)

Ooi, C.H., et al.: Physiological characteristics of elite and sub-elite badminton players. J. Sport. Sci. **27**(14), 1591–1599 (2009)

Phomsoupha, M., Laffaye, G.: The science of badminton: game characteristics, anthropometry, physiology, visual fitness and biomechanics. Sports Med. **45**(4), 473–495 (2015)

Potteiger, J.A., et al.: Muscle power and fibre characteristics following 8 weeks of plyometric training. J. Strength Cond. Res. **13**, 275–279 (1999)

Rathore, M.S.: Effects of plyometric training and resistance training on agility of tennis players. Indian J. Phys. Educ. Sport Med. Exerc. Sci. **16**(1 & 2), 32–34 (2016)

Salonikidis, K., Zafeiridis, A.: The effects of plyometric, tennis-drills, and combined training on reaction, lateral and linear speed, power, and strength in novice tennis players. J. Strength Cond. Res. **22**(1), 182–191 (2008)

Seiler, S., Joranson, K., Olesen, B.V., Hetlelid, K.J.: Adaptations to aerobic interval training: interactive effects of exercise intensity and total work duration. Scand. J. Med. Sci. Sport. **23**, 74–83 (2013)

Sloth, M., Sloth, D., Overgaard, K., Dalgas, U.: Effects of sprint interval training on VO2max and aerobic exercise performance: a systematic review and meta-analysis. Scand. J. Med. Sci. Sport. **23**, 341–352 (2013)

Walklate, B.M., O'Brien, B., Paton, C.D., Young, W.B.: Supplementing regular training with short-duration sprint agility training leads to a substantial increase in repeated sprint-agility performance with national level badminton players. J. Strength Cond. Res. **23**(5), 1477–1481 (2009)

Wee, E.H., Low, J.Y., Chan, K.Q., Ler, H.Y.: Effects of high intensity intermittent badminton multi-shuttle feeding training on aerobic and anaerobic capacity, leg strength qualities and agility. In: Proceedings from icSPORTS 2017: The 5th International Congress on Sport Sciences Research and Technology Support. Science and Technology Publications, Lisbon (2017)

Ziemann, E., Olek, R., Grzywacz, T.G.A.: Aerobic and anaerobic changes with high-intensity interval training in active college-aged men. J. Strength Cond. Res. **25**(4), 1104–1112 (2011)

Criteria of Individualization of Short Distance Runners Training

Anna Zakharova[✉] and Tatiana Miasnikova

Institute of Physical Education, Sport and Youth Policy,
Ural Federal University named after the first President of Russia B.N. Yeltsin,
19 Mira Street, 620000 Yekaterinburg, Russia
sport_tsp@mail.ru, tmyas@yandex.ru

Abstract. To achieve high sports results it is important to determine the individual structure of athlete preparedness. Information about specific preparedness of short distance runner may be a tool of training management and individualization. The transience of sprint competitive activity actualizes the use of support technologies for the search of informative criteria. Nine male short distance runners aged 17–22 were recruited for the study. Along with the pedagogical tests (vertical jumps and 30 m running) modern measurement equipment and software ("Neurosoft" (Ivanovo, Russia), the MED BIKE ergometer (Technogym, Italy) and Cardio Memory software V 1.0 SP3) were used to obtain data on various indicators of specific preparedness of sprinters.

The study of individual characteristics of advanced short distance runners revealed significant differences in the structure of specific preparedness among athletes. Evaluation of the relationship between objective indicators of the psychophysiological, functional and morphological properties of athletes and results of competitive activity was the basis for establishing the criteria of training individualization of short distance runners.

Keywords: Short distance runners · Training and testing ·
Criteria of individualization

1 Introduction

The principle of individualization of training [6] is a priority in the training of well-trained athletes. Another important factor in achieving high athletic results is to focus training on the specific features of the competitive activity.

Sprint requires an elementary forms of speed qualities (latent reaction time, movement frequency and speed) and their complex forms, characterizing the level of development of power qualities (peak power, speed and strength endurance etc.). The majority of these indicators may be improved only through high-intensity work performing. Then using of physical loads of this intensity level (without taking into account individual peculiarities of the athlete) can provoke the exhaustion of adaptive resources, which will not allow to achieve high performance [2, 4, 5, 7, 10, 12]. So only the information about the preparedness structure and individual features of the sprinter can be a tool of training management and individualization.

© Springer Nature Switzerland AG 2019
J. Cabri et al. (Eds.): icSPORTS 2016/2017, CCIS 975, pp. 204–212, 2019.
https://doi.org/10.1007/978-3-030-14526-2_14

As sprint running is extremely fast it is hard to evaluate the structural components of performance without use of modern information technologies. This situation actualizes the search of informative criteria to assess the individual specific preparedness of short distance runners with the use of athletes' testing support technologies in order to provide individualization of training [14].

2 Organization and Methods

Research Organization. The research was conducted in Ural Federal University in 2016. Nine advanced short distance runners (males, age 19.9 ± 2.1 years; the level of sports results: 60 m running – 6.8–7.1 s; 200 m running – 21.0–22.5 s) took part in the research. The participants of the study had more than 7 years of sport experience in track-and-field. All subjects were free of cardiovascular or any other chronic disease. The investigation conforms to the principles of the Declaration of Helsinki of the World Medical Association. Athletes had been provided with comprehensive information on the procedures, methods, benefits and possible risks involved in the study before their written consent was obtained. The study was approved by the Ural Federal University Ethics Committee [14].

Informative indicators to identify the structure of the training of short distance runners in the study were determined in the process of measuring and analyzing test results of components specially trained group of sprinters with the use of modern measuring equipment and technologies:

- software complex "Neurosoft" (Ivanovo, Russia) for measuring and assessing physiological characteristics of athletes (speed – latent reaction time, movement frequency);
- the MED BIKE ergometer (Technogym, Italy) and Cardio Memory software V 1.0 SP3 is to measure peak power, speed-power qualities, power endurance;
- biodynamic evaluation of muscle composition [11] – to estimate biodynamic muscle composition.

For the assessment of psychophysiological features of athletes the hardware and software complex "Neurosoft" (Ivanovo, Russia) was used. Two tests were conducted with "Neurosoft" in the research: simple sensomotor reaction (SSMR) and Tapping test. Following indicators were defined in SSMR: average time of 30 attempts of reaction, number of signal omissions (SO) and early reaction (ER).

Tapping test (rapid tapping with electronic stick on electronic plate during 30 s) was conducted for finding of nervous processes strength by monitoring of tapping rate dynamics in every five seconds interval. Total amount of taps (TA), taps frequency, workability graph character with taps distribution in 5 s intervals were under consideration.

Cycling Wingate test was conducted with the use of the ergometer BIKE MED (Technogym, Italy) and Cardio Memory software V 1.0 SP3. The athlete has 30 s to perform the leg cycling at maximum speed with load, which is set automatically in accordance with the athlete body weight. Anaerobic power measures were obtained using leg cycling Wingate anaerobic test, and included peak power (PP, W), relative PP (W/kg), power at 15 s (P_{15}, W) and 30 s (P_{30}, W), average power (AP_{30}) and their relative values (P_{15}, W/kg, P_{30}, W/kg, AP_{30}, W/kg) and fatigue (F, %).

Maximum vertical jump test involves the execution of a standing countermovement vertical jump with hands on hip with fixing its height. Subjects were asked to perform three attempts with a recovery interval sufficient for the realization of the maximum potential of athletes in each attempt.

The determination of maximal jump height testing was done with video recorder camera. Between the camera and athlete transparent ruler – a sheet of plexiglass with nontransparent transverse graduations was installed [11]. It allows to fix the maximum height of an athlete waist belt control marker movement. Once jump testing is complete, the video was viewed frame-by-frame on the monitor. Thus the determination of the jump height and time of peak height reaching of the waist marker were proceeded.

The repeated jump test was also used in the proposed set of short-distance runner tests to define biodynamic evaluation of muscle composition [11]. The athlete performed 40–50 maximal (all-out) standing countermovement vertical jumps.

The percentage indicator of slow twitch muscles content K was calculated according to a formula: height during the test was carried out through video as in maximum jump test in our research:

$$K = H_{30} \div H_{max} \times 100\% \tag{1}$$

where H_{30} – average height of the thirty first, thirty second and thirty third jumps, H_{max} – average height of the first three vertical jumps [11].

Statistical analysis was performed with the use of statistic software package Microsoft Excel. Mean value (M) and standard deviation (SD) of the used parameters were calculated.

For each studied parameter three levels were set:

– the average level with indicators being in range $M \pm 0.5$ SD;
– above the average with indicators more than $M + 0.5$ SD;
– below the average with indicators less than $M - 0.5$ SD [13].

For a holistic understanding of the level of athletes specific physical preparedness each athlete's result was rated in accordance with established levels: below the average – 1, the average – 2 and above the average – 3.

3   Results and Discussions

3.1   Using MED BIKE Ergometer (Technogym, Italy) for Cycling Wingate Test in Short Distance Runners Testing

The rates that are fixed when you pedaling in the regime of Wingate test allow to analyze the structure of the power abilities of athletes (Table 1). There are two types of main power characteristics – absolute and relative power of performing the pedaling and the degree of fatigue that are derived on the monitor during the test.

Table 1. Wingate test results (M ± SD) and structure of power level in short distance runners.

Indicators	M ± SD	The levels of indicators of power (point)								
		A1	A2	A3	A4	A5	A6	A7	A8	A9
Peak power, W	861 ± 84	2	3	3	2	1	3	1	3	2
Power at 15 s, W	769.1 ± 71.7	2	3	2	2	2	2	1	3	2
Power at 30 s, W	562.9 ± 77.4	2	3	1	2	1	2	3	2	3
Average power, W	722.9 ± 71.1	2	3	2	2	1	2	1	2	2
Relative peak power, W/kg	11.9 ± 1.3	1	1	3	2	1	3	1	3	1
Relative power at 15 s, W/kg	10.6 ± 1.2	1	1	2	2	1	3	1	3	1
Relative power at 30 s, W/kg	7.7 ± 0.8	1	3	1	3	1	2	3	3	2
Average relative power, W/kg	9.9 ± 0.9	1	2	3	3	1	3	2	3	2
Power reduction, %	36.7 ± 5.9	2	3	1	3	2	2	1	1	3
The sum of scores for the absolute power	–	8	12	8	8	5	9	6	10	9
The sum of scores for the relative power	–	4	7	9	10	4	11	7	12	6
Total score	–	12	19	17	18	9	20	13	22	15
The overall level of speed-power development	–	1	2	2	2	1	3	1	3	2

A1-9 athletes, 1 point – below average, 2 points – average, 3 points – above average.

Analyzing the obtained results, it can be noted that the structure of speed-power abilities of athletes differ from each other. So, athlete 6 has the highest relative power and a high level of absolute power during the test in comparison to other athletes. The athlete 2 with high level of absolute power over the entire test showed a low level of relative power in the first half of the test. The structure of speed-power abilities in the athlete 5 is significantly different: he has a low level of all indicators of relative power and most of the indicators of absolute power.

To assess the speed-strength endurance level we analyzed the degree of fatigue and the dynamics of relative power during performing Wingate test (Table 2).

In the analysis of the power dynamics of Wingate test (Table 2) it is important to consider its initial level, because in case of low initial level its decline is less pronounced, so the fatigue level will be lower. But we are interested of higher power that may be kept up as long as possible.

The Technogym computer calculates the fatigue degree taking into account PP, P_{min} and time between them. As a result the degree of fatigue by Technogym is hard-to-explain (the second column of Table 2). In our research and in sport practice we use the power decline rate (columns 3–6). For example, dynamics of the power of A7 with the lowest peak power was the lowest. However, his level of fatigue was assumed high by Technogym.

The analysis of the power decline rate in athletes showed (1) great differences in advanced sprinters: from 15.5 (A7) to 46.5% (A3); (2) power reduction was non-linear: more intense in the second half (12.5–35.9%) than in the first half (3.4%–17.5%).

Table 2. Dynamics of power indicators of sprinters during performing the Wingate test.

Athletes	Fatigue degree, % (BIKE MED Technogym)	Relative peak power, W/kg	$\Delta W_{max} - W_{15c}$, %	$\Delta W_{15c} - W_{30c}$, %	$\Delta W_{max} - W_{30c}$, %	The level of power endurance
1	39	10.54	17.5	27.1	39.8	2
2	27	10.91	5.4	19.3	23.6	3
3	42	13.09	16.5	35.9	46.5	1
4	34	12.30	9.4	24.2	31.3	3
5	37	11.14	12.2	29.4	38.0	2
6	38	13.14	11.7	34.5	42.1	2
7	43	10.39	3.4	12.5	15.5	3
8	42	14.15	10.4	33.3	40.3	1
9	28	11.14	5.1	27.3	31.0	3
Average	36.7	10.6 ± 1.1	10.2	27.1	34.3	

1 – below average, 2 – average, 3 – above average.

Individual structure of indicators dynamics must output prompt how to correct training: either pay more attention to leg muscles hypertrophy in case of low level of peak power or to devote more time to speed and strength endurance in case of great fatigue degree or poor Wingate test finish power.

3.2 Using of Jump Tests to Assess Components of the Specific Preparedness in Short Distance Runners

Two jump tests included in the set of tests for assessing specific fitness level of sprinters, were used to estimate explosive power and the percentage of slow fibers in muscles of legs (Table 3). The innate ratio of fast and slow twitch muscles is one of the important factors of achieving success in sprint. Olympic Champions in sprint are characterized by a predominance of type II motor units (or fast twitch fibers), the content of which is up to 60%.

Table 3. The explosive power and leg muscles composition of short distance runners.

Indicators	M ± SD	A1	A2	A3	A4	A5	A6	A7	A8	A9
Vertical jump height, cm	52.2 ± 3.7	3	3	3	2	2	3	1	1	1
Content of slow twitch muscles, %	67.2 ± 7.8	3	2	2	2	2	2	2	2	1

Results of repetition maximal test revealed the relatively low content of slow twitch motor units indicating the high level of potential development of power only in one athlete (A1). On the contrary athlete 9 (A9) has a high percentage of slow twitch motor units, that is a low potential in sprinting. The rest of the athletes are within the average, that means that they need corrections in the training process in favor of increasing the volume of exercises aimed at developing power or extend the competition distance length [1, 8, 9].

3.3 Use of Psychophysiological Tests for the Nervous System Strength Assessment

Performing psycho-physiological tests (Tapping-test and SSMR) allowed us to estimate speed of latent sensomotor reaction, signal omissions (SO), early (premature) responses (ER) (Table 4) and type of the nervous system (Fig. 1). Analysis of the results of the tapping test and SSMR indicates significant performance differences among the athletes (Table 4).

Table 4. Psychophysiological status of short distance runners.

Indicators	M ± SD	A1	A2	A3	A4	A5	A6	A7	A8	A9
Total amount of taps	207.1 ± 25.3	2	2	2	2	1	2	3	3	2
SSMR, ms	143.6 ± 12.7	2	3	3	2	1	3	1	1	3
SO	1.4 ± 0.9	1	1	1	2	1	2	2	3	2
ER	2.9 ± 2.5	1	1	2	3	1	3	2	3	2

SSMR – simple sensomotor reaction, SO – the number of signal omission, ER – the number of early responses.

There are three types of the nervous system: strong, weak and intermediate [3]. The results of tapping test was used to determine the type of the nervous system of sprinters (Fig. 1).

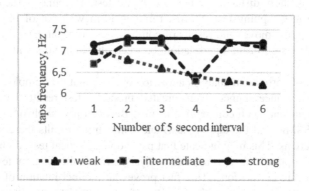

Fig. 1. Tapping test workability graph of sprinters with different types of nervous system [14].

According to the results of tapping-test all types of nervous system in sprinters were revealed: strong nervous system with even workability of athletes (A1, A3, A8), weak with the descending graph (A4, A5, A7) and an intermediate type (A2, A6, A9).

Type of athlete nervous system revealed in tapping-test in our study was seen as the key to the physical load distribution in a workout: for athletes with strong type of nervous system the physical load can be distributed evenly in the main part of training session. An intermediate type is characterized by reduced performance in the middle of work and its restoration to baseline levels after short period of "rest" (frequency fall-off) in tapping test. So, for effective training session the physical load, especially in high-intensity programs, should be divided in two or three parts to det the most out of the workouts. In case of downward type of workability intensive work should be carried out in the first half of the training sessions [14].

The importance of latent reaction is undeniable in sprint. The norm of reaction in the sprint disciplines is considered to be in the interval from 120 to 150 ms for high performance sport athletes. Most of the participants of the study showed the result of SSMR within the athlete norm that confirms their availability for sprint running. As well as increased frequency of taps (more than 200 per 30 s) serves the indicator of ability to perform high intensity physical load. "Neurosoft" (Ivanovo, Russia) provides data of signal omissions and premature responses that usually are not analyzed. These indicators give us important information on the psychophysiological state of the athlete. Premature reactions in SSMR test may indicate potential for good results in sprint, and omissions, on the contrary, their absence.

3.4 The Interrelation Between the Components of the Specific Preparedness of Short Distance Runners

Each test used in the study provide the researcher with a large number of indicators, but not all of them have the same importance. For using them in training management it is necessary to identify the most reliable, meaningful and informative indicators.

Correlation analysis between 17 indicators obtained as a result of tests for specific preparedness of short distance runners (Wingate test, maximal vertical jump test, repeated jump test, tapping test, SSMR, running 30 m with out of blocks start and running 30 m on the move) and results of competitive activity in the 60 m and 200 m running revealed significant interrelation between the indicators only in five tests (Table 5).

The results of correlation analysis allow to conclude that the complex of suggested tests for short distance runners were created properly: test results have significant correlation coefficients with competitive results. Between psychophisiological tests by "Neurosoft" (SSMR and the tapping-test) and competitive results there were not significant connections. This may indicate that psychophisiological tests do not reflect the specifics of sprint, but further correlation analysis between the different tests indicators revealed significant correlations. That fact proves an indirect relation of psychophysiological indicators and competition results of sprinters. The results of these psychophisiological tests can be used for improvement of the organizational aspects of the training (sport selection, physical load distribution, etc.).

Correlation analysis between the 17 indicators of different tests against each other showed that there is a low unreliable connection between the indicators of the tests. It is supposed that the result of each test separately characterizes the level of one components of the specific preparedness of athletes in sprint thus it points to the necessity of

Table 5. Correlation of the indicators of tests for special preparedness assessment and competitive results of short distance runners.

Test	Indicators	Correlation factor	
		60 m running time	200 m running time
Cycling Wingate test	Peak power	−.601*	−.303
	Relative Peak power	−.423	−.614*
Maximum jump test	Vertical jump height	−.688*	−.545
Repeated jump test	Vertical jump height changing	.719*	.646*
·30 m running with out of blocks start	Running time	.872**	.682*
30 m running on the move	Running time	.654*	.791**

* − p < 0.05, ** − p < 0.01

using not a single test, but their complex for integral characteristics of specific preparedness. Significant correlation (P < 0.01) was detected only in four cases: between the indicators of the degree of fatigue in Wingate test and signal omissions (r = −0.79) and early responses (r = −0.85) in SSMR test; between the results of maximum vertical jump and the percentages of slow twitch muscles from the repeated vertical jump test (r = −0.94); between the average reaction time in the SSMR-test and the result in running 30 with out of block start (r = −0.78). The obtained correlation results indicate the need for inclusion of psychophysiological tests in tests complex for sprinters specific preparedness assessment.

4 Conclusions

1. The main criteria for training design and individualization of advanced athlete training should be (1) specific to the competitive activity and (2) objective to reflect psychophysiological, functional and morphological properties of the athlete. Criterial indicators should give an adequate assessment of the athlete's condition and allow to identify the strengths and weaknesses of preparedness.
2. The assessment of specific preparedness of short distance runners must include following tests: Wingate test, maximal vertical jump test, repeated jump test, tapping test, SSMR, running 30 m with out of blocks start and on the move. This tests complex should be upgraded by psychophysiological tests.
3. The research of individual athlete characteristics of advanced short-distance runners highlighted the significant differences in the structure of athletes' specific preparedness, their strengths and weaknesses that must be taken into account during training design.

Acknowledgements. The work was supported by Act 211 Government of the Russian Federation, contract # 02.A03.21.0006.

References

1. DeWeese, B., Hornsby, G., Stone, M., Stone, M.: The training process: planning for strength–power training in track and field. Part 1: theoretical aspects. J. Sport Health Sci. **4** (4), 308–317 (2015)
2. DeWeese, B., Hornsby, G., Stone, M., Stone, M.: The training process: planning for strength–power training in track and field. Part 2: practical and applied aspects. J. Sport Health Sci. **4**(4), 318–324 (2015)
3. Ilyin, E.: Methodical instructions to the workshop on psychophysiologyю Leningrad (1981)
4. Kenney, L., Wilmore, J., Costill, D.: Physiology of Sport and Exercise, Human Kinetics, 6th edn. Human Kinetics Publishers, Champaign (2015)
5. Kuznetsova, Z., Kuznetsov, A., Mutaeva, I., Khalikov, G., Zakharova, A.: Athletes preparation based on a complex assessment of functional state. In: Proceedings of the 3rd International Congress on Sport Sciences Research and Technology Support, pp. 156–160. SCITEPRESS (2015)
6. Matveev, L.: The General Theory of Sport and Its Applied Aspects. Soviet sport, Moscow (2010)
7. Myakinchenko, E., Seluyanov, V.: Development of Local Muscle Endurance in Cyclic Sports. TVT-Division, Moscow (2009)
8. Platonov, V.: System of Training Athletes in Olympic Sports. The General Theory and Its Practical Applications. Olympic literature, Kiev (2004)
9. Seluyanov, V.: Preparation of Middle Distance Runner. TVT-Division, Moscow (2007)
10. Shephard, R., Astrand, P.-O.: Factors to be measure. In: Endurance in Sports. COPYRIGHT, pp. 271–272. International Olympic Committee (2008)
11. Shishkina, A.: Biodynamical estimation of human muscle composition. In: Uchenye zapiski universiteta imeni P.F. Lesgafta, vol. 45, no. 11, pp. 108–111 (2008)
12. Verkoshansky, Y.: Programming and Organization of the Training Process. Fizkultura and Sport, Moscow (1985)
13. Zaciorskij, V.: Sports Metrology. Fizkultura and Sport, Moscow (1982)
14. Zakharova, A., Miasnikova T.: Individualization of short distance runners training based on analysis of specific. In: Proceedings of the 5th International Congress on Sport Sciences Research and Technology Support: icSPORTS, vol. 1, pp. 115–120 (2017)

Author Index

Printed in the United States
By Bookmasters